Breastfeeding Telephone Triage and Advice

3rd Edition

Maya Bunik, MD, MSPH, FABM, FAAP

American Academy of Pediatrics Publishing Staff

Mary Lou White, *Chief Product and Services Officer/SVP, Membership, Marketing, and Publishing*

Mark Grimes, *Vice President, Publishing*

Peter Lynch, *Senior Manager, Digital Strategy and Product Development*

Leesa Levin-Doroba, *Production Manager, Practice Management*

Jason Crase, *Manager, Editorial Services*

Mary Louise Carr, *Marketing Manager, Clinical Publications*

Published by the American Academy of Pediatrics

345 Park Blvd

Itasca, IL 60143

Telephone: 630/626-6000

Facsimile: 847/434-8000

www.aap.org

The American Academy of Pediatrics is an organization of 67,000 primary care pediatricians, pediatric medical subspecialists, and pediatric surgical specialists dedicated to the health, safety, and well-being of infants, children, adolescents, and young adults.

The recommendations in these protocols do not indicate an exclusive course of treatment or serve as a standard of medical care. Variations, taking into account individual differences and circumstances, may be appropriate.

Statements and opinions expressed are those of the authors and not necessarily those of the American Academy of Pediatrics.

Products and Web sites are mentioned for informational purposes only and do not imply an endorsement by the American Academy of Pediatrics. Web site addresses are as current as possible but may change at any time.

Brand names are furnished for identification purposes only. No endorsement of the manufacturers or products mentioned is implied.

Every effort has been made to ensure that the drug selection and dosages set forth in this text are in accordance with the current recommendations and practice at the time of publication. It is the responsibility of the health care professional to check the package insert of each drug for any change in indications and dosages and for added warnings and precautions.

Some drugs and medical devices presented in this publication have US Food and Drug Administration (FDA) clearance for limited use in restricted research settings. It is the responsibility of health care professionals to ascertain the FDA status of each drug or device planned for use in their clinical practice.

This publication has been developed by the American Academy of Pediatrics. The contributors are expert authorities in the field of pediatrics. No commercial involvement of any kind has been solicited or accepted in development of the content of this publication.

Every effort is made to keep *Breastfeeding Telephone Triage and Advice* consistent with the most recent advice and information available from the American Academy of Pediatrics.

Special discounts are available for bulk purchases of this publication. E-mail Special Sales at aapsales@aap.org for more information.

Printed in the United States of America

9-294

1 2 3 4 5 6 7 8 9 10

MA0870

ISBN: 978-1-61002-197-5

eBook: 978-1-61002-198-2

Cover design by Wild Onion Design

Library of Congress Control Number: 2017962656

To my beloved breastfed children, Larissa, Marko, and Nick.

Nursing each of you was the truest of blessings and the highlight

of working motherhood for me.

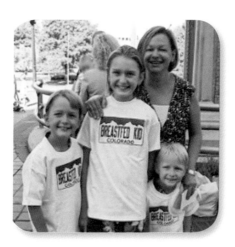

Acknowledgments to the Third Edition

- As with previous editions, to my patients, families, and colleagues for their contributions to the new color photographs here.

- **Lorry Watkins, RN, IBCLC,** my clinical partner in my consultative breastfeeding practice, for her help with obtaining color photos and consents.

- **Robin Pence, RN,** an amazing nurse in my primary care clinic and photographer, for her photoediting.

- **Dr Mary O'Connor** of the Executive Committee of the Section on Breastfeeding for her review of this third edition, as well as for her continued support across the miles.

Acknowledgments to the Second Edition

- **Dr Joan Meek,** Chair of the American Academy of Pediatrics Section on Breastfeeding, and triage nurse leaders Teresa Hegarty and Kelli Massaro for their thorough and thoughtful reviews of this second edition.

- **Dr Dena Dunn** for important additional photographs and for being an invaluable psychologist and colleague of the Trifecta Approach for Breastfeeding Management.

- **John Babiak** for assistance with photoediting.

- **Peter Lynch,** editor, for his guidance with this second edition.

Acknowledgments to the First Edition

I would like to thank Barton Schmitt, MD, FAAP, for giving me the template to write this companion book to *Pediatric Telephone Protocols*. Writing this book with his guidance was a true professional gift. I continue to enjoy and learn working alongside him clinically at our primary care clinic at Children's Hospital Colorado.

I am grateful to

- **Stephen Berman, MD, FAAP,** past American Academy of Pediatrics (AAP) president, who was instrumental in helping me return to Colorado and launching my academic career. He has been the best career mentor I could ever wish for.

- **Marianne Neifert, MD, FAAP,** who has been an excellent career-long mentor for me and planted the seed about the rewards of helping mother-baby pairs with breastfeeding back in the late 1980s. She has inspired and advised me over the years with my advocacy and research projects.

- **Nancy Hilton, MD,** my first Ambulatory Division head at Children's Hospital & Research Center Oakland, who realized that not only did our clinic need breastfeeding expertise, but I needed a clinical niche and sent me to my first physicians' joint AAP and La Leche League International (LLLI) breastfeeding conference in 1998 in Santa Fe.

- **Benjamin Gitterman, MD, FAAP,** who, along with other great career and life advice, told me to get involved in the AAP.

- **Allison Kempe, MD, MPH, FAAP,** my outstanding research mentor, with whom I wrote my first breastfeeding research grant. She continues to guide my work and writing.

- Lactation consultants in California who helped me start the breastfeeding residency curriculum and taught me so much about breastfeeding management along the way: **Laura Monin, IBCLC; Fritzi Drosten, RN, IBCLC;** and **Joanne Jasson, RN, IBCLC.**

- **Maryann Kerwin,** one of the founders of LLLI, who continues to inspire me with her positive approach to legislation challenges and the difficulty supporting working breastfeeding mothers in our economy; and **Cate Colburn-Smith** and **Jennifer Dellaport,** the 2 other "musketeers" of the Colorado Breastfeeding Coalition, with whom I share the passion and commitment of helping Colorado mothers with breastfeeding.

- **Mary O'Connor, MD, MPH, FAAP,** my current codirector of the resident breastfeeding curriculum, who I met "on the Internet" looking for online learning programs for my residents while I was in Oakland.

- Lactation Consultant **Lorry Watkins, RN, IBCLC,** my amazing clinic partner in breastfeeding management faculty practice at Children's Hospital Colorado, who reviewed the clinical content of this book; and **Beth Gabrielski, RN, IBCLC,** and **Jeannine Hoelskin, RN, IBCLC,** for all their teaching and support.

- St. Louis group—**Randy Sterkel, MD, FAAP,** and **Isabel Rosenbloom, MD, FAAP; Suzi Wells, RN; Pam Flotte, RN; Lisa Swerczek, RN; Christine Lune, MSN, CPNP;** and **Diane Williams, RN**—for their thorough and thoughtful reviews.

- **Kathie Marinelli, MD, IBCLC, FABM, FAAP,** and **Bonny Whalen, MD, IBCLC,** who did rigorous and relevant reviews and are not only my Academy of Breastfeeding Medicine colleagues but have become dear friends.

- Pediatric after-hours nurse leaders **Teresa Hegarty** and **Kelli Massaro** for their triage expertise and critique of final drafts of this book. Also, nurses **Sharon Palmer** and **Betsy Bridges** from Children's Medical Center practice who provided invaluable input from an office-based perspective.

- **Richard Schanler, MD, FAAP, chair,** and the AAP Section on Breastfeeding leadership team for their expert review.

- **Diane Della Maria, AAP editor,** for her kind and steady guidance over the past year.

- **Maria Barrera,** our family's first caregiver for 6 years, who supported my breastfeeding relationships with my children and was careful not to waste any precious human milk. She helped me return to work after my first baby, which was such a critical period.

- My professional mother-friends, **Lisa Kremer, MD; Nancy Showen, MD; Laura Grunbaum, MD, FAAP; Yasmin Carim, MD, FAAP; Liz Walser, MSW; Debra Bogen, MD, FAAP;** and **Jenny Kempe-Biermann, MD,** who shared the journey of breastfeeding and working motherhood with me.

- **Jennie** and **Rob Dawe** and their girls, who shared so many wonderful moments and photographs with me for this book.

- My breastfeeding patients—all the mother-baby pairs and their families who bring me the privilege of helping them; the "intimacy among strangers" is such a part of this work. I am also grateful for their willingness to be photographed in clinic. As a nursing mother and family medicine physician, **Kelly McMullen** understood the need for certain photographs and went above and beyond with assisting me.

- My sister, **Tania Bunik,** for her technical assistance with the photos and for continuing to share the journey of motherhood with me.

- My family—children **Larissa, Marko, and Nick,** and husband **John**—who supported me through many long weekends while I was writing this book.

- Finally, my father **Peter Bunik** for always reminding me that "Maya, I Believe in You!" and the late **Nina K. Bunik,** for choosing to nurse me during a time in the early 1960s when women were being encouraged to "take a medicine to dry up breast milk" and formula-feed. She was there for my daughter Larissa's first latch after birth and stayed for 6 weeks. What a blessing to have had my dear Mama's support as a new mother.

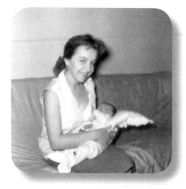

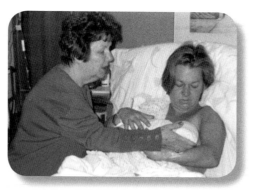

Preface and How to Use This Book

Breastfeeding Telephone Triage and Advice is to be used in the context of a healthy mother-baby dyad. It is written for nurses, lactation professionals, and other staff in doctors' offices who triage breastfeeding questions by telephone or offer advice. This book should be used as a companion to *Pediatric Telephone Protocols* by Barton D. Schmitt, MD, FAAP.

Newborns are a high-risk group because congenital diseases and serious infections can present in the first few weeks after birth. As stated by Dr Schmitt, "Feeding behavior is one of the universal and reliable measures of a newborn's well-being." **At any time, if the health care professional triaging or providing advice has any concerns, the baby should be referred for urgent evaluation, recognizing that poor feeding or a change in feeding behavior can be a symptom indicating serious illness.** Other symptoms of illness in a newborn besides poor feeding include poor or weak suckling; sweating with feedings; sleeping excessively; change in muscle tone; decrease in activity; change in color; fever or low temperature; unusual crying, moaning, or grunting; and tachypnea.

My goal here is to make triage and advice as straightforward, formatted, and evidence-based as possible. However, managing breastfeeding is an art. It requires sensitivity to the intimacy involved and significance to the mother. This respectfulness is as important as the science—deciphering the symptoms and determining the best course of action for the problem while being careful to not disrupt the delicate balance that is the breastfeeding dyad.

Maya Bunik, MD, MSPH, FABM, FAAP

Reference
Schmitt BD. *Pediatric Telephone Protocols: Office Version.* 16th ed. Itasca, IL: American Academy of Pediatrics; 2019

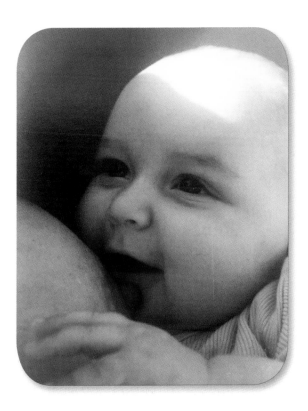

Breastfeeding Support in the Office Setting

(Adapted from Bunik M. The pediatrician's role in encouraging exclusive breastfeeding. Pediatr Rev. 2017;38[8]:353–368.)

If you have acquired this book for your office or hospital staff, you are to be commended, as this is a good step toward creating a breastfeeding friendly and knowledgeable environment.

In my breastfeeding consultative practice, I spend much of the visit guiding mothers and families through the many questions they have generated from searching the Internet. I anticipate that this third edition of the book helps you to serve parents better during this vulnerable time in the early months with feeding their new baby. It is so rewarding to be their informed guide.

Some suggestions for supporting breastfeeding in the office setting include

- Evaluate early and often in first 3 to 4 weeks when breastfeeding is getting established.

- Address combination feeding: Early supplementation with formula can adversely affect the feeding duo and is a risk factor for early cessation.

- Advocate for maternity leave and support the mother's often stressful return-to-work transition/milk storage and child care communication suggestions (see protocols).

- Train office staff or provide early referral to a known lactation specialist for breastfeeding management and support.

- Provide resources for mothers, such as hospital-based drop-in clinics and/or other mother support groups. It is always a good idea to attend, or have one of your office staff attend, these sites so that you are sure that the advice and any concerns raised are addressed appropriately and in line with general American Academy of Pediatrics recommendations.

- Avoid storing or giving out formula samples in your office. It may seem supportive, but it gives the wrong message about breastfeeding exclusivity. Providing information about pumps, pump rental stations, or videos on hand expression is a better idea.

Additional Items to Consider Providing

- Hospital-grade pump not only to assess whether mother's single use pump is effective but to assess milk supply status in your office (baby just fed or mother unsure)

- Breastfeeding pillow

- Area in waiting room designated with sign "Breastfeeding Welcome Here"

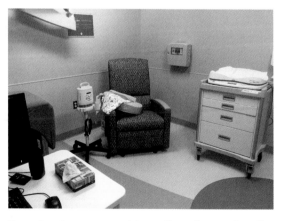

Examination room with recliner, breastfeeding pillow, breast pump, and scale set up.

Alphabetic Contents

Alphabetic Contents (continued)

Topic Contents

Topic Contents (continued)

Baby, Later

Special Circumstances

Appendixes

Triage Assessment Questions

When using these advice topics, it is best to begin each call with the following 10 screening questions and then ask, "What is your main breastfeeding question or concern?"

Screening Questions for Early Postpartum Period—First 2 Weeks

❶ **What is your baby's age and gestation? Was your baby born early or on time? If early, how early? Do you have discharge sheets at home? Did the hospital tell you your infant's gestational age?** (Late preterm is high-risk.)

❷ **Is your baby acting sick or abnormal in any way (eg, weak, decreased activity)?** *R/O sepsis, particularly in babies 4 weeks and younger*

❸ **Is breastfeeding going well?** If not perceived as going well, mother and baby may need to be seen in the office today or tomorrow (within 24 hours).

❹ **How many times have you breastfed in the past day?** Optimal is 10 to 12 times per 24 hours; minimum of 8 times. Suboptimal nursing sessions require evaluation.

❺ **How long is your baby awake and actively suckling and swallowing at the breast during a feeding?** Baby should be actively feeding at the breast without long pauses or flutter feeding for at least 10 minutes. Just as with microwave popcorn, pauses or extended time (ie, cooking it too long) is not effective (analogy courtesy of Sheela Geraghty, MD, MS, IBCLC, FAAP). Mother may need assistance with latch and keeping baby on task for nursing sessions.

❻ **What color are your baby's stools?** By day 4, stools should be yellow and seedy, not black or green transition stools.

❼ **How many stools has your baby had in the past day?** Goal is 1 per day after birth up to day 4 (ie, by day 4, should have at least 4 stools). Suboptimal stool pattern requires evaluation.

❽ **How many wet urine diapers?** Usually 7 to 8 wet urine diapers (exception: 3 wet diapers per day can be normal in first 5 days). Suboptimal urine pattern requires evaluation.

❾ **Do your breasts feel full before feedings and softer afterward?** Optimal answer is yes. Before milk is in, most mothers will not notice any change. If baby is close to 2 weeks of age, mother's breasts may be adjusting to what the baby's needs are, and she may experience only mild symptoms of engorgement.

❿ **How many times have you supplemented with formula in the past day?** Supplementation more than once in 24 hours can affect milk supply or may indicate breastfeeding difficulties.

Adapted from Screening Form for Early Follow-up of Breastfed Newborns. Dr. Mom Web site. http://www.dr-mom.com. Copyright © 2012 Marianne Neifert, MD, MTS. Reproduced with permission.

Copyright © 2019 Maya Bunik, MD, MSPH, FABM, FAAP

ALCOHOL USE (MOTHER)

Definition

Alcohol transfers readily into human milk according to the mother's blood alcohol level. Peak levels usually are seen within an hour of ingestion.

TRIAGE ASSESSMENT QUESTIONS

Go to ED Now

● Symptoms of irritability or sedation in baby
Reason: evaluation of baby for alcohol intoxication

Home Care

○ Mother ingested one drink—glass of wine (5 ounces), beer (12 ounces), or cocktail (1.5 ounces of 80 proof)—and feels unaffected.

○ Mother ingested more than the safe limit of one drink in 2 hours.

HOME CARE ADVICE

❶ **Single "Celebratory" Alcoholic Beverage:** An occasional glass of wine (5 ounces), beer (12 ounces), or cocktail (1.5 ounces of 80 proof) is acceptable. You should nurse first, have the drink, and then wait at least 2 hours. If you feel affected by the drink and your breasts feel uncomfortably full, you should pump and dump the milk.

❷ **Drinking in Excess:** If you want to drink more, you should pump and dump for at least 8 hours or until you no longer feel affected by the alcohol. Waiting about 2 hours per drink is required for complete metabolism of alcohol in a 180-pound woman. Once your blood level is down, your milk level is also down and, therefore, safe for your baby. Only time eliminates alcohol from your system; drinking water or caffeine, exercising, or pumping more does not work.

❸ **Test Strips for Alcohol:** Because some mothers cannot self-assess if they feel affected, test strips are growing in popularity. Hand-expressed drops of milk can be placed on the strip, or the strip can be dipped into a small sample of human milk. Milkscreen home test for alcohol in breast milk (available at Target, Walmart, and Amazon) detects the presence of alcohol at 13.1 mg/dL or greater in human milk.

BACKGROUND INFORMATION

- It is well-known that alcohol is hazardous to the fetus in pregnancy.
- If careful, the mother can consume alcohol in moderation without harm to her nursing baby.
- Low-level drinking during breastfeeding is not associated with shorter breastfeeding duration or adverse developmental outcomes in infants at 12 months.
- Heavy drinking by the mother (more than one drink in 2 hours) may affect the ability to safely care for her baby.
- Alcohol inhibits oxytocin release and the letdown process while it is in the mother's bloodstream, so suggestions that drinking beer can enhance milk supply are incorrect (previously, the yeast and barley in home brew was felt to be a galactagogue).

ALLERGY (SPECIAL CIRCUMSTANCES)

Definition

- Variety of symptoms attributed to intake of milk, such as eczema, rash, or hives; wheezing; congestion; red, itchy eyes; irritability or colic; vomiting; constipation or diarrhea; or green stools with mucus or blood.
- Current evidence does not support maternal dietary restrictions during pregnancy and lactation, even for peanuts or tree nuts.

TRIAGE ASSESSMENT QUESTIONS

See Other Protocol

- Fussiness, Colic, and Crying in the Breastfed Baby on page 41
- Spitting Up (Reflux) on page 96
- Gassiness in the Breastfed Baby on page 44

See Within 3 Days in Office *(by Appointment)*

- Baby having any symptoms or signs suspicious of allergy, such as eczema, rash, or hives; wheezing; congestion; red, itchy eyes; irritability or colic; vomiting; constipation; or diarrhea
  Reason: possible allergy to a substance transmitted in mother's milk, such as bovine milk proteins
- Any blood or mucus in stools
  Reason: possible allergy
- Family history of allergies
  Reason: possible allergy
- Extremely fussy most of the time, not just during late afternoon and evening hours as with more traditional or usual colic periods
  Reason: possible allergy
  Caution: Conclusions about allergy to dairy should not be made over the telephone because many of these symptoms can occur with other conditions. Dairy allergy occurs in only 2 to 3 of 100 babies. If mother continues to be concerned about possible allergic cause, she can bring diaper or stool sample to an office visit to be tested for blood.

Home Care

- ○ Trial elimination of dairy from mother's diet

HOME CARE ADVICE

❶ **Dairy Suspicion:** If you feel strongly about dairy as cause of symptoms in your baby,
- First eliminate drinking milk.
- If no improvement with milk elimination, next eliminate all milk products, including cheese and ice cream, for 2 weeks to see if it causes any change in your baby's behavior or symptoms.
- Read ingredients of all food products and avoid products that contain milk powder, casein, or whey (all of which can be found in many prepared foods).
- These diets are difficult to maintain and can be associated with unnecessary early breastfeeding cessation.

❷ **Call Back If:** Your baby seems sick, or home care advice is not helping.

BACKGROUND INFORMATION

- Allergy symptoms in a baby who ingests human milk when the mother has ingested bovine milk, artificial colors or preservatives, eggs, wheat, chocolate, or nuts.
- Food hypersensitivity is not immunoglobulin E mediated (not anaphylaxis).
- Human milk has been found to be protective, or at least may delay presentation, of allergic manifestations of eczema, wheezing, asthma, and allergies.
- Usually occurs in the context of a family history of food allergies, but not always.

BITING BREAST, ONSET AT 6 MONTHS (BABY, LATER)

Definition

- Infant biting at breast when breast is offered or at the end of a feeding when nursing is finished.
- Infant cannot bite and drink milk at the same.

TRIAGE ASSESSMENT QUESTIONS

See Other Protocol

- Nursing Strike or Refusal on page 84
- Sore Nipples on page 93

See Today or Tomorrow in Office (by Appointment)

- Breast or nipple wound from bite that looks infected
  Reason: may need antibiotics

Home Care

- ○ Infant biting at beginning of feed
  Reason: infant offered breast but not hungry
- ○ Infant biting at end of feed
  Reason: infant finished with feeding

HOME CARE ADVICE

❶ **Disengage Biting Infant:** Make sure your infant comes off quickly from the breast. Biting needs to be addressed immediately.

❷ **Indicate Firmly, "No Biting":** Touch your infant on the lips and say, "No biting." If you reacted by screaming or crying, your infant may have received the message. Some infants even refuse to go to the breast for a short period (see Nursing Strike or Refusal on page 84).

❸ **"Disappear":** You should quickly set your infant down in a safe place and leave the room.

❹ **Anticipate Possible Biting During Future Feedings:** An infant needs to be hungry for nursing. Once finished, your infant needs to come off quickly.

❺ **Watch for Infection:** If bite breaks the skin, watch the bite mark on the breast closely because of increased risk of infection.

❻ **Call Back If:** Advice not helping. See within 3 days in office (by appointment).

BACKGROUND INFORMATION

- Prior to 6 months of age, crying or fussing was associated with hunger but now may indicate just wanting to be held or played with. Putting the older infant to the breast when not hungry is not uncommon and sorting out this transitional period can be challenging.
- Simultaneous tooth eruption may cause the infant to exhibit teething behaviors and make him more likely to bite.

BREAST MASS (MOTHER)

Definition

Lump or change in the breast that does not improve with nursing or pumping (Plugged ducts and mastitis are the most common reasons for breast mass.)

TRIAGE ASSESSMENT QUESTIONS

Go to ED Now *(or to Office With PCP Approval)*

● Fever, chills, or feel systemically ill
Reason: if mastitis, may need treatment with oral antibiotics or hospitalization for intravenous antibiotics

See Other Protocol

● Breast Pain (for mastitis and plugged duct) on page 6
● Color Change of Human Milk on page 16

See Today or Tomorrow in Office *(by Appointment)*

● Localized redness on skin surface or tenderness of breast
● Pain with palpation
Reason: if mastitis, may need antibiotics

See Within 3 Days in Office *(by Appointment)*

● New lump
R/O fibrocystic disease versus other mass
● Rubbery mass
R/O lipoma versus other mass
● Soft and squishy or feels as if it is fluid filled
R/O galactocele
● Lumpy and tender breasts all over
R/O fibrocystic disease of breast, granulomatous mastitis
Reason: not sure mother can discern these aspects of lump, so presence of any new lump necessitates evaluation and may need ultrasound or biopsy

Home Care

○ Localized tender cord of tissue
R/O plugged duct
○ Lump that improves with pumping
R/O plugged duct
○ History of trauma to the breast, inflammation, bruising, or hematoma in breast tissue

HOME CARE ADVICE

❶ **Pain Control:** You may take ibuprofen (eg, Advil, Motrin); because of its anti-inflammatory properties, it is the best choice for pain. Acetaminophen (eg, Tylenol) can be added if needed. Both medications are compatible with nursing.

❷ **Plugged Ducts**
- **Warm Comfort:** Try a warm pack (eg, hot water bottle, barley pack that can be put in microwave for this use) on the plugged duct site prior to feeding or pumping.
- **Massage:** Apply direct pressure to the breast, pushing thickened area toward the nipple (almost pushing it out) while your baby is feeding there or while manually or electronically expressing milk.
- **Lecithin:** Some clinicians recommend soy lecithin for plugged ducts, but no research studies support use of this herbal preparation. Soy lecithin is a naturally occurring fatty acid and available in capsule or liquid form. Dose is 1 tablespoon of granules once daily or 1 to 2 capsules (1,200 mg each) 3 to 4 times a day.
- **Good-Fitting Bra:** Be sure to wear a good-fitting supportive bra; areas of tightness can impede milk flow.
- **Trauma of the Breast:** If history of breast trauma, bruising hematoma or fat necrosis may be associated. These should all resolve with time.

❸ **Call Back If:** Advice not helping. See within 3 days in office (by appointment).

BACKGROUND INFORMATION

Causes

- **Solid Tumor:** Fibroadenoma, including ectopic breast adenomas (axilla, chest wall, vulva); lipoma.
- **Post-mastitis Abscess.**
- **Papilloma:** Benign epithelial tumor.
- **Fibrocystic Disease:** Hormonally mediated benign proliferation of alveolar system with variable degrees of pain, tenderness, and palpable thickening or nodules.
- **Granulomatous Mastitis:** Usually presents as mastitis or a breast mass and requires a biopsy for diagnosis; usually requires anti-inflammatory drugs, such as prednisone or methotrexate, for treatment (very rare).
- **Galactocele:** Benign cystic tumor containing milk or a milky substance in the breast caused by a protein plug that blocks off the outlet; may be associated with oral contraceptive use.
- **Inflammation Due to Trauma, Hematoma.**
- **Fat Necrosis:** Benign condition that consists of fatty tissue that has been bruised or injured in the breast.
- **Cancer:** Should be considered in persistent breast masses, but it is reassuring that only 3% of those with diagnosed breast cancer are pregnant or lactating.

BREAST PAIN (MOTHER)

Definition
Pain of the larger breast area not confined to nipple region

TRIAGE ASSESSMENT QUESTIONS

Go to ED Now *(or to Office With PCP Approval)*
- ● Fever, chills, or feel systemically ill
  Reason: if mastitis, may need treatment with oral antibiotics or hospitalization for intravenous antibiotics

See Other Protocol
- ● Sore Nipples (for Raynaud disease of the nipple/vasospasm) on page 93
- ● Breast Mass on page 4
- ● Engorgement on page 25

See Today or Tomorrow in Office *(by Appointment)*
- ● Localized redness on skin surface, generalized tenderness of breast, or both
  Reason: may mistake these symptoms for engorgement and may not be able to self-assess to rule out mastitis adequately
- ● Pain with palpation
  Reason: if mastitis, will need outpatient antibiotics

See Within 3 Days in Office *(by Appointment)*
- ● Nipples or areolar area pink, shiny, or flakey
  R/O yeast infection
- ● Shooting (from nipple to back) or burning pain
  R/O yeast infection
- ● Maternal antibiotics at time of delivery
  R/O yeast infection
- ● Mother prone to yeast infections
  R/O yeast infection
- ● Maternal diabetes
  R/O yeast infection
- ● Chronic breast tenderness despite treatment with antibiotics or antifungals
  R/O bacterial infection of lactiferous ducts or coexisting bacterial and candidal infections
- ● Eczema-like appearance to nipples or skin over breast (dry, red, itchy)
  R/O eczema

- ● Exposures to irritant (eg, soaps, laundry detergent with dye/fragrance)
  R/O contact dermatitis
- ● Unilateral nipple that looks as if it has eczema
  R/O Paget disease

Home Care
- ○ Feeling of fullness or hardness to both breasts
  R/O engorgement
- ○ One-sided, localized pain to a specific area within breast
  R/O plugged duct
- ○ Palpable lump or cord of tissue
  R/O plugged duct

HOME CARE ADVICE

❶ **Pain Control:** You may take ibuprofen (eg, Advil, Motrin); because of its anti-inflammatory properties, it is the best choice for pain. Acetaminophen (eg, Tylenol) can be added if needed. Both medications are compatible with nursing.

❷ **Comfort Measures:** Cold pack can be placed on breasts for comfort.

❸ **Pain With Letdown:** Some clinicians recommend evening primrose oil, an herbal preparation that is rich in alpha-linolenic acid, although no research studies support its use.

❹ **Engorgement Suspected**
- **Frequent Feedings:** Breastfeed approximately every 2 hours (10–12 feedings in 24 hours). If you are too uncomfortable to breastfeed or your baby cannot latch on because of engorged breasts, express milk manually or with a hand or mechanical pump at least every 3 hours (but more frequently if able).
- **Warm Comfort:** Taking a warm shower or placing a warm washcloth on breasts before nursing may help get milk flowing.
- **Cold Comfort:** More severe engorgement may require cool compress, such as a gel or an ice pack. Refrigerated, raw, clean cabbage leaves may also provide relief because of their coolness and ability to shape around the breast.

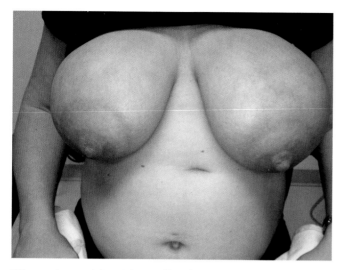

Bilateral mastitis with swollen breasts and erythema

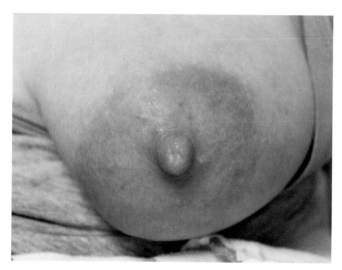

Raynaud disease/vasospasm blanching of nipple after nursing

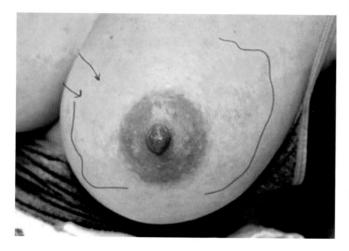

Mastitis can be subtler with erythema and induration, outlined here in black.

- **Reverse-Pressure Softening Technique:** Gentle 2-handed pressure on the breast to push edema away from the areola may help your baby latch better.

❺ Plugged Duct Suspected
- **Warm Comfort:** Try a warm pack (eg, hot water bottle, barley pack that can be put in microwave for this use) on the plugged duct site prior to feedings or pumping.
- **Massage:** Apply direct pressure to the breast, pushing thickened area toward the nipple (almost pushing it out) while your baby is feeding at the breast or while manually or electrically expressing milk.
- **Lecithin:** Some clinicians recommend soy lecithin for plugged ducts, but no research studies support use of this herbal preparation. Soy lecithin is a naturally occurring fatty acid and available in capsule or liquid form. Dose is 1 tablespoon of granules once daily or 1 to 2 capsules (1,200 mg each) 3 to 4 times a day.
- **Good-Fitting Bra:** Be sure to wear a good-fitting supportive bra; areas of tightness can impede milk flow.

❻ Check Pump Settings: If pumping ensure that suction settings are at a comfortable level. Many mothers assume that "max" level is better.

❼ Call Back If: Advice not helping. See within 3 days in office (by appointment).

BACKGROUND INFORMATION

Causes
- **Engorgement:** Fullness and pain of the breast. In the first few days of milk coming in, the fullness is related to increased milk production but also to edema and increased vascularity. After this time, engorgement is most often associated with inadequate drainage of the breast from infrequent feedings (eg, mother-baby separation, a sleepy baby) or a poor latch.
- **Plugged Duct:** Collection of ducts in the breast gets blocked temporarily by inadequate drainage of milk, resulting in a small, painful, thickened area of the breast. Occasionally, calcium stones may be the cause.

- **Mastitis:** Pain and redness of the breast that is often associated with systemic symptoms of fever, chills, and body aches. If pain and tenderness are prolonged, abscess should be considered.
- *Candida* **(Yeast) Infection:** Shooting sensation from a mother's nipple to her back or a burning-type pain has most often been associated with a yeast infection. With *Candida* infection, the mother may also have a pink- or red-tinged nipple area with some peeling and shininess to the surrounding skin. Several recent studies have been unable to culture yeast in the milk of mothers with this type of pain, having cultured staph and strep instead, raising the question of whether the pain may be from another condition.
- **Paget Disease:** A superficial manifestation of underlying breast malignancy appearing as a small vesicular eruption with persistent soreness, pain, or itching of the nipple or areola.
- **Pain With Letdown:** Combination of higher levels of prolactin and lower levels of alpha-linolenic acid.
- **Teen Mothers:** These mothers initiate breastfeeding but commonly stop due to pain. Referral to see a lactation specialist for support may be warranted.

Treatment Options

Note: Treatment for these conditions is usually empiric and not diagnosed by culture methods.

- **Mastitis Suspected:** Cephalexin/dicloxacillin or clindamycin if methicillin-resistant *Staphylococcus aureus* (MRSA) is suspected. MRSA is emerging as a cause of mastitis. Case reports have shown that with MRSA, mothers have less pain and fever, and these low-grade symptoms result in delayed care and treatment and increased risk of abscess formation.
- *Candida* **Infection Suspected:** Nystatin cream for the mother's nipples, or oral fluconazole (100–200 mg daily for a few weeks), and simultaneous baby treatment with oral nystatin or gentian violet.

BREAST PAIN, CHRONIC >1 WEEK (MOTHER)

Definition

Pain of the larger breast area not confined to nipple region lasting longer than 1 week or not improving with treatment

TRIAGE ASSESSMENT QUESTIONS

Go to ED Now (or to Office With PCP Approval)

● Fever, chills, or feel systemically ill
Reason: if mastitis, may need treatment with oral antibiotics or hospitalization for intravenous antibiotics

See Other Protocol

● Sore Nipples (for Raynaud disease of the nipple/vasospasm) on page 93

See Today or Tomorrow in Office (by Appointment)

● Localized redness on skin surface or tenderness of breast
● Pain with palpation
Reason: if mastitis, may need outpatient antibiotics; pain is a common cause of weaning, so it should be evaluated urgently

HOME CARE ADVICE

❶ **Pain Control:** You may take ibuprofen (eg, Advil, Motrin); because of its anti-inflammatory properties, it is the best choice for pain. Acetaminophen (eg, Tylenol) can be added if needed. Both medications are compatible with nursing.

❷ **Comfort Measures:** Cold pack can be placed on breasts for comfort.

❸ **Check in About Breast-Pump Trauma:** Check for proper flange fit (only a small portion of areola should move into flange space); avoid excessive high pressure or sessions of prolonged duration (not >20 minutes).

BACKGROUND INFORMATION

Causes

- Pain and redness of the breast that is often associated with systemic symptoms of fever, chills, and body aches may be mastitis. If pain and tenderness are prolonged, abscess or staphylococcal infection should be considered.
- Staphylococcal infections are thought to be the most common etiology, so oral treatment may need to be adjusted to address one.
- Dermatoses such as eczema, psoriasis, or Paget disease can cause persistent pain and become secondarily infected.
- Allodynia or functional pain is a rare cause, and mothers usually have a history of pain disorder such as fibromyalgia or irritable bowel syndrome.

BREASTFEEDING IN THE FIRST FEW WEEKS: SIMPLIFY YOUR LIFE (ADVICE ONLY) (BABY, EARLY)

TRIAGE ASSESSMENT QUESTIONS

See Other Protocol

● Fathers (Advice Only) on page 31

Here is home care advice that may be offered to any mother calling about issues in the first few weeks of her breastfeeding experience.

Dear New Mother,
You should
- Live as if you are on a vacation. That means
  - Do not house clean.
  - Do not do laundry; live as if you are staying at a hotel or condominium (eg, live out of a suitcase, buy extra socks and underwear for you and your partner).
  - Eat off paper plates.
  - Get creative about meals: accept offers from others, make dinner in the morning when you are less tired, and get takeout or semi-homemade meals (eg, supermarket roasted chicken and ready-made mashed potatoes).
- Minimize entertaining (ie, avoid visits that involve being a hostess for guests who come to admire your baby). This can wait until after the first month.
- Wait to write thank-you notes and make phone calls. Post a message on Facebook or on your front door, or record a message on voice mail: "We are adjusting to the new addition to our family. We would love to see you in a month when we are more rested and settled."
- Remember that naps are crucial. Naps without your baby in the building need to be planned with your partner or spouse and extended family. Have someone take your baby out for a few hours so you can get carefree sleep—sleep without hearing every snort and funny baby breathing sound your baby may make. Some mothers may actually sleep better if their baby is nearby. If this is the case for you, just remember to lie down and try to sleep whenever your baby is sleeping!

- Try to stay in bed for a few days, in your pajamas, and just breastfeed your baby. This usually does wonders for your milk supply.
- Create a nest and have a basket in the same area with diapers, wipes, breast pads, a water bottle, snacks, and other personal items, such as a phone.

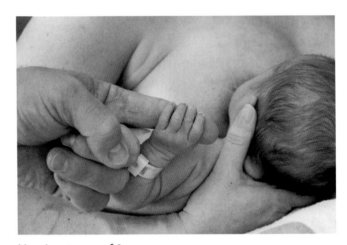

Nursing team of 3

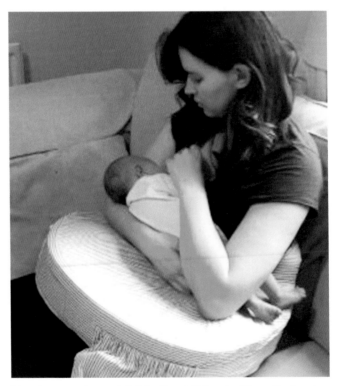

Nursing mother with My Brest Friend pillow that acts like a shelf

BREASTFEEDING STATION SUPPLIES (ADVICE ONLY) (MOTHER)

GENERAL CONSIDERATIONS

Here is the list of supplies you need for your breast-feeding journey.

- Good-fitting nursing bra.
- Cotton cloth nursing or disposable pads if prone to leaking milk.
- Lanolin cream.
- Pick a comfortable location. Your preference may be for a private spot versus a central location in the home (isolated in a faraway room may be less desirable).
- Large or comfortable chair (eg, sofa chair, glider rocker, La-Z-Boy chair). Sometimes the glider or other rocking chairs can be too snug for a breast-feeding pillow.
- Footstool or ottoman.
- Side table for supplies.
- Special breastfeeding pillows, such as a Boppy, can be used to wrap around you and your baby. Some mothers prefer bed pillows for support. My Brest Friend has a "shelf effect."
- Water in refillable bottle and drinking to satisfy thirst.
- Healthy snacks or meals nearby.

- Breastfeeding uses 500 calories per day. Replenish with healthy foods by making and storing in the refrigerator (eg, smoothies, premade pasta salad) when hungry. Have a ready-made snack close by on the side table (eg, fruit, granola bar); eat to satisfy hunger.
- If pumping, activities such as watching a favorite program or recorded show or reading a magazine or book can assist with motivation. A hands-free nursing bra is helpful for pumping. Keeping your baby nearby may help with letdown.
- If a sibling is involved, it is a good idea to have a special bin of books, stickers, and other activities that come out only when nursing. Siblings can be encouraged to help by tickling the baby's feet to keep her on task with feeding. Drawing attention to the special time set aside for the older sibling by announcing in a dramatic voice, "Now it is Mom (or Dad) and _____ (insert child's name here) time!" may help with sibling rivalry.

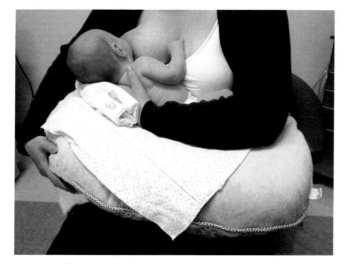

Boppy pillow to support baby during feeding

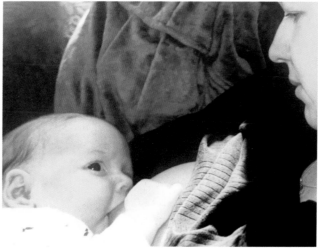

A comfortable chair/location is preferred.

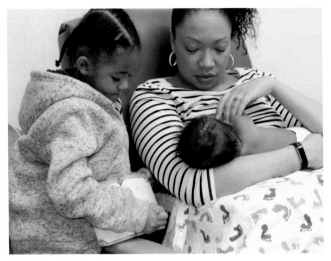

Older sibling drawing in close proximity to mother-baby pair

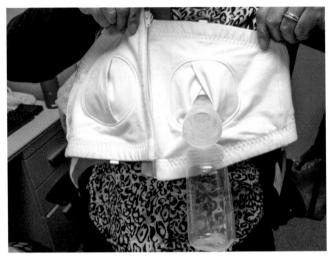

Hands-free pumping bra

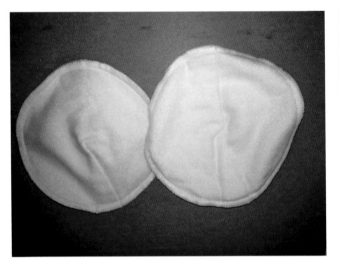

Cotton breast pads

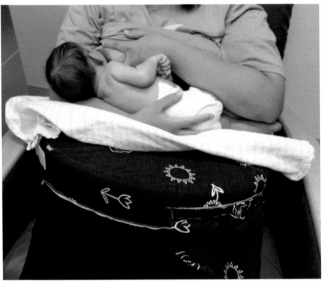

Mother and baby nursing at their breastfeeding station in a central place in the home

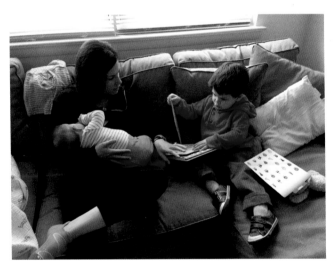

Sibling enjoys a special activity in close proximity to mother and baby nursing.

CHILD CARE AND BREASTFEEDING (ADVICE ONLY) (SPECIAL CIRCUMSTANCES)

GENERAL CONSIDERATIONS

- Child care facilities should support mothers on the breastfeeding journey by ensuring that staff are trained to handle human milk, follow mother's feeding plan, and understand the judicious use of pumped milk.
- Child care staff should provide good communication about schedules and milk volumes and allow a quiet place for working mothers to nurse on-site. For example, a mother may want to nurse as she re-unites with her baby at the end of the working day before driving home together.
- Data from the Infant Feeding Practices Study showed that breastfeeding at 6 months was significantly associated with support from child care providers.
- Model breastfeeding policy is provided at the CGBI: National Collaborative for Advancing Breastfeeding in Child Care Web site (https://sph.unc.edu/cgbi/national-collaborative-on-advancing-breastfeeding).
- Helpful resource: *Breastfeeding in Child Care Toolkit* (http://county.pueblo.org/sites/default/files/documents/Breast%20Feeding%20in%20Child%20Care%20Toolkit%28Centers%29_1.pdf).

The 10 Steps for Baby-Friendly Child Care

Step 1: Have a written policy that reflects the program's commitment to promoting and supporting breastfeeding, especially exclusive breastfeeding, and share with employees and families.

Step 2: Train and evaluate all staff in the skills to support and promote optimal infant and young child feeding.

Step 3: Inform women and families about the importance of breastfeeding.

Step 4: Provide learning and play opportunities that normalize breastfeeding for children.

Step 5: Ensure that all breastfeeding families are able to properly store and label their breast milk for child care use.

Step 7: Support breastfeeding employees.

Step 8: Ensure that each infant has a feeding plan that supports best feeding practices.

Step 9: Contact and coordinate with community breastfeeding support resources.

Step 10: Train all staff (teaching and nonteaching) annually on the protection, promotion, and support of breastfeeding.

CLICKING OR NOISY NURSING (BABY, EARLY)

Definition
Clicking, snorting, or other upper airway noises heard with nursing at the breast

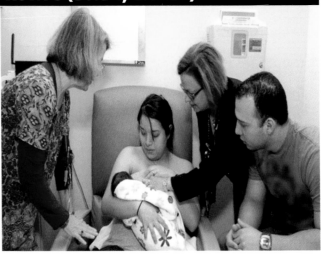

Early evaluation of noisy nursing is key.

TRIAGE ASSESSMENT QUESTIONS

See Other Protocol
- Sore Nipples on page 93
- Tongue-tie on page 102
- Overactive Letdown/Overabundant Milk Supply on page 86

See Today or Tomorrow in Office *(by Appointment)*
- Ask mother to describe sound. Most noises are due to faulty latch and will sound like clicking or smacking.
- Tongue has notch or is heart shaped
  R/O tongue-tie
- Baby's tongue does not protrude or retract out with crying
  R/O tongue-tie
- Latch is painful
  Reason: concern for tongue-tie and may need referral to trained provider (surgeon, dentist, neonatologist, otolaryngologist) who performs frenotomy
- Sound is associated with increased work of breathing
  Reason: may need to R/O hypoxia, possible laryngomalacia, or other anatomic abnormality

See Within 3 Days in Office *(by Appointment)*
- Continued noisy feeding, coming off the breast frequently
- Continued sore nipples and not improving
- Overactive letdown not improving
  Reason: may need evaluation by lactation expert

Home Care
- ○ Sounds like congestion or stuffy nose
- ○ Choking or crying with feeding
  R/O overactive letdown

HOME CARE ADVICE

❶ **Noisy Feedings:** Most noises are caused by faulty latch. To achieve a good latch, ensure that your baby has a wide mouth, upper and lower lips flared, chest to your abdomen, and knees and legs wrapped around your body.

❷ **Bulb Syringe Suction:** A baby with a stuffy nose may benefit from saline suction of nasal passages.

❸ **Nipple Pain or Maternal Frustration With Feedings:** Pump until referral can be made for latch evaluation.

❹ **Overactive Letdown/Overabundant Milk Supply:** Consider feeding in a leaning-back position and breastfeeding on only one side each feeding. This can help with downregulating milk supply.

BACKGROUND INFORMATION

Causes

- **Faulty Latch:** Main cause of noisy nursing.
- **Response to Fast Flow:** Babies may alter suck to respond to rapid letdown or faster flow when nursing.
- **Short Frenulum:** Of newborns, 2% to 5% have tongue-tie at birth. It can be familial, may affect latch, and is a common cause of clicking.
- **Upper Airway Obstruction:** Nasal passages may have congestion and result in noisy nursing.
- **Laryngomalacia:** Floppy airway that collapses on itself.
- **Palate Abnormality:** More usual to have a subtle palate abnormality. Babies with true cleft lip and palate usually have difficulty achieving latch.
- **Retracted Jaw or Tongue.**
- **Congenital Micrognathia (Small Jaw) or Pierre Robin Sequence:** Anatomically difficult for tongue to come forward.

COLOR CHANGE OF HUMAN MILK (BABY, EARLY)

Definition

- Blood-tinged or pinkish watery discharge also known as rusty-pipe syndrome.
- Baby has pink-tinged spit-up related to this symptom.
- Other colors of human milk, such as orange, green, pink/red, and black, can be related to certain medications or food substances.

TRIAGE ASSESSMENT QUESTIONS

Go to ED Now (or to Office With PCP Approval)

- ● Fever, chills, and feel systemically ill
  Reason: mastitis likely and may need hospitalization for intravenous antibiotics

See Other Protocol

- ● Breast Mass on page 4
- ● Sore Nipples on page 93
- ● Breast Pain (for mastitis) on page 6

See Today or Tomorrow in Office (by Appointment)

- ● Discharge or milk that looks like pus
  Reason: infection
- ● Fever
  Reason: infection
- ● Symptoms that present longer than a few weeks
  Reason: intraductal papilloma (small, harmless tumors of milk ducts), possible cancer, or other breast mass

Home Care

- ○ Discharge or milk watery and pink or orange in color
  R/O rusty-pipe syndrome, use of breast pump at high settings, or older infant going through growth spurt who may be nursing more rigorously
- ○ Cracking or sores on nipples that could be bleeding
  R/O sore nipples
- ○ Maternal contraceptives, tranquilizers
  R/O medication adverse effect
- ○ Maternal medications or food sources
  R/O adverse medication or food color effect

HOME CARE ADVICE

1. **Rusty-Pipe Syndrome:** Cause is increase in blood vessels and expansion of milk ducts. Continue feeding. You may see blood come out in stool, but the blood is not dangerous to your baby; this should fade in a week or so. If your baby is older, the trauma of capillaries may occur with rigorous pumping or strong suckling during a growth spurt.

2. **Sore Nipples (With or Without Cracking/ Bleeding)**
   - **Pain Control:** You may take ibuprofen (eg, Advil, Motrin); because of its anti-inflammatory properties, it is the best choice for pain.
   - **Lanolin and Hydrogel/Soothies Pads:** If you have sore nipples, you should keep your nipples covered with a medical-grade pure lanolin ointment and a hydrogel dressing, or Soothies Gel Pads, which will encourage cracks to heal without scabbing or crusting. (These supplies can be found at Target and Babies"R"Us, respectively.) To cool them, place on a clean plate in the refrigerator while nursing. Mini–ice packs can be made out of 4" × 4" gauze and freezing in a reusable, resealable storage bag in freezer. Tea bags, formerly a folklore remedy, are no longer recommended because the tannic acid in the tea is an astringent and can cause drying and cracking.
   Note: No need to wash lanolin off nipples.

3. **Review of Medications:** Various colors can be an adverse effect of medications. For example, green with iron or propofol, red with rifampin, and black with minocycline. Check with your doctor or pharmacist.

4. **Review of Foods:** Ingested food dyes can affect milk color—orange or yellow from carotenoids in carrots or yellow vegetables, pink/red from beets, and green from green vegetables.

5. **Call Back If:** Your baby is acting sick or advice is not helping. See within 3 days in office (by appointment).

BACKGROUND INFORMATION

- This is usually benign if it occurs late in pregnancy or in first few weeks postpartum. It is rare later on. It is transient and caused by a large increase in blood vessels and expansion of milk ducts.
- Occurs in 15% of asymptomatic women and usually fades in 3 to 7 days.
- Usually presents as red- or brownish-colored milk associated with blood from cracked or sore nipples.
- Mother becomes concerned because she notices pink-tinged emesis.
- An unusual color in mother's milk can cause worry too, but it is usually a benign cause.

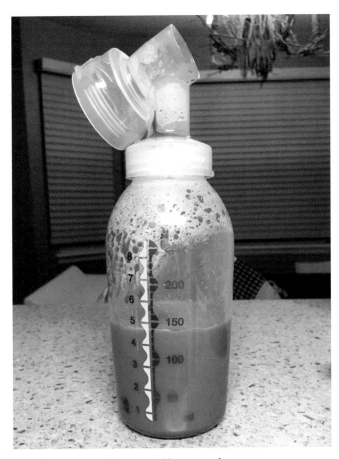

Blood-tinged milk caused by use of pump at too high settings

CONSTIPATION IN THE BREASTFED BABY (BABY, LATER)

Definition

- Pain or crying with the passage of a hard stool or inability to pass a stool.
- In a breastfeed infant, this usually happens when the infant is older than 1 month.

TRIAGE ASSESSMENT QUESTIONS

See Other Protocol

⬤ Fussiness, Colic, and Crying in the Breastfed Baby on page 41

⬤ Gassiness in the Breastfed Baby on page 44

See Today in Office *(by Appointment)*

⬤ Breastfed newborn younger than 1 month, may be a sign of poor intake

⬤ Infant 1 to 2 months and suspected not normal straining and grunting
  R/O congenital causes (eg, anal stenosis, Hirschsprung disease, hypothyroidism, infection due to botulism)

See Within 3 Days in Office *(by Appointment)*

⬤ Breastfed infant older than 1 month and continued suppository use

⬤ Small bleeding from anal fissure

Home Care

○ Infant grunting or straining with stooling

○ Breastfed infant 4 to 8 weeks of age with more prolonged period without a stool; no vomiting or discomfort
  R/O breastfed stool variant

○ Changes in breastfed infant's diet (eg, addition of formula or baby or solid foods)

HOME CARE ADVICE

❶ **Normal Grunting and Straining:** It is normal for babies to grunt and strain with stools, even in older babies for brief periods. They feel and experience their stools more dramatically.

❷ **Breastfed Stool Variant:** About one-third of breastfed babies can have one soft and voluminous (ie, "large blowout") stool every 4 to 12 days (longer stretches can occur but are rarer). Longer periods yield larger stools. Being prepared with a change of clothes, blankets, and diaper wipes is important because cleanup can be an ordeal due to overflow and leakage.

❸ **Constipation From Recent Changes in Diet**

- For babies older than 1 month, add 1 ounce of apple or pear fruit juice per month of age per day.
- For babies on solid/baby foods, add higher fiber foods, such as peas, beans, apricots, prunes, peaches, pears, and plums.
- Try keeping your baby's legs in a flexed position.
- A warm bath relaxes stomach muscles, and your baby may pass stool in the tub.
- Glycerin suppository (over the counter) inserted into the rectum can help because it acts as an anal lubricant and mild osmotic stimulant, bringing fluid into the stool so it can pass easier. If glycerin suppositories are being used frequently, your baby should be evaluated.

❹ **Call Back If:** Advice not helping. See within 3 days in office (by appointment).

BACKGROUND INFORMATION

Causes

- Stooling pattern depends on adequate human milk intake and age of a baby; expect one for each day after birth up to day 4, and then stools every feeding or every other feeding for the first few weeks. In early days, colostrum in the breastfed baby acts as a natural laxative to move meconium and darker green transition stools.
- Decreased stooling in breastfed newborns younger than 1 month may indicate inadequate intake.
- Slow intestinal transit time.
- Using occasional formula supplementation or combination feeding with human milk can cause constipation and typically occurs when an infant is older than 1 month.
- Addition of baby foods at 6 months or older.
- **Breastfed stool variant at 4 to 8 weeks of age** occurs in about one-third of breastfed infants, who can have one soft and large stool blowout every 4 to 12 days (longer can occur but is rarer) because of almost complete absorption of human milk.

CONTRACEPTION, LACTATION AMENORRHEA METHOD (ADVICE ONLY) (MOTHER)

GENERAL CONSIDERATIONS

Common Questions

- I have heard that not having my menstrual period when nursing is enough protection against pregnancy. Is this true?
- Can contraception affect my milk supply?
- What are the best choices for contraception when I am breastfeeding?

  Note: An exhaustive list of contraceptive brand names is not included here so the information stays basic. For more information, the triage practitioner is encouraged to use the resources listed in References on page 111.

Amenorrhea Method

- This method of contraception relies on every-3-hour nursing throughout the 24-hour period for ovulation to be reduced.
- It has 3 necessary components.
  - Baby is younger than 6 months.
  - Menstrual period has not returned.
  - Mother is fully or nearly fully breastfeeding (ie, no formula, no complementary feeds) during the day with at least one feeding through the night.
- With this frequency of nursing, amenorrhea is common in the first 6 months of nursing and is associated with only a 2% chance of pregnancy.
- This can be reduced to 1% if combined with basal thermal temperature and cervical mucus secretion monitoring for timing of the fertile period (and avoiding sexual intercourse during this period).
- If baby has started taking longer stretches of sleep at night (ie, ≥4 hours), an alternative method of contraception is recommended if mother does not desire to become pregnant.

Contraceptive Agents

- Low-dose progestin only (eg, Nor-QD) is the best choice for minimal effect on milk volume and weight gain in baby. Some mothers can be sensitive to even progesterone only; therefore, it is recommended that mothers try progesterone pills first before obtaining an injection or intrauterine device (IUD).
- Progesterone IUD (eg, Mirena) or vaginal rings with progesterone initially appeared safe but recently have been reported to decrease milk volume in some women.
- Progesterone implants (eg, Norplant) or injections (eg, Depo-Provera) may also have an effect on milk volume and weight gain in a baby.
- Barriers are nonhormonal and so do not affect lactation but are less likely to be effective in preventing pregnancy (eg, male/female condoms are only 82% effective; cervical cap, 88% effective).
- Combined estrogen/progestin should be avoided because of risk of lower milk volume and, therefore, slower weight gain in baby.

COSLEEPING/BED SHARING AND BREASTFEEDING (ADVICE ONLY) (BABY, EARLY)

Definition

Cosleeping means that parent and baby are in close proximity in same room but not the same contiguous surface together when asleep. Bed sharing, sleeping on the same surface, is a form or subset of cosleeping but is not recommended by the American Academy of Pediatrics because of risk of unintentional suffocation.

BACKGROUND INFORMATION

Causes

- In 2006, sudden infant death syndrome (SIDS) was found to be related to issues with sleep arousal centers in the brain and babies' response to hypoxia.
- In 2007, a genetic link or relationship was found to associate long QT syndrome with SIDS.
- SIDS is a sudden and unexplained death of a seemingly healthy infant in the first year after birth. SIDS most commonly occurs in infants aged 2 to 4 months and is rare before 1 month or after 6 months of age.
- Non-SIDS causes of infant death include child abuse, such as abusive head trauma (formerly known as shaken baby syndrome); suffocation or overlaying; birth defects; metabolic abnormalities; and infection.

Cosleeping/Bed Sharing Issues

In many cultures, cosleeping and bed sharing is common.

- Twenty-two percent of parents of 1-month-olds report bed sharing, and up to 40% report bed sharing overall in the United States.
- Babies who bed share breastfeed 3 times longer than those who do not, but emphasis should be given to safe cosleeping practices and prevention noted in the Home Care Advice section.

HOME CARE ADVICE

❶ **Note Message:** The American Academy of Pediatrics has expressed concern about bed sharing. Better to put your baby back to sleep for every sleep in a separate space in close proximity to you (parents) or in a bassinet or cosleeper close to the bedside. It is recommended that they sleep in the parents' room ideally for the first year but at least for the first 6 months.

❷ **Close by for Convenience:** When babies are sleeping close by but in a separate space, it is easier to reach for them to nurse during the nighttime.

❸ **Select Bedding Carefully:** Babies should be on a flat, firm surface, with no padding, bumpers, quilts, duvets, comforters, or lambskins.

❹ **Avoid Adult Beds:** Especially waterbeds, recliners, and sofas.

❺ **Avoid Sedating Substances:** You (parents) or caregivers should avoid alcohol, cigarette smoking, and sedating drugs or medication. Do not bed share if you use any of these substances, even if it is prescribed medication, because of increased risk of overlaying.

❻ **Avoid Overheating:** Keep room temperature moderate and avoid over-bundling your baby. Swaddling is not recommended as a strategy to avoid SIDS. Once a baby shows the ability to roll, swaddling should be discontinued.

❼ **Consider Pacifier Use:** Pacifier at last sleep has been associated with decreased risk of SIDS, but the mechanism is unclear. Routine use of pacifiers in the first month after birth is not recommended for the breastfed infant until breastfeeding is well established.

❽ **Avoid Others in Bed:** No pets or other children in bed.

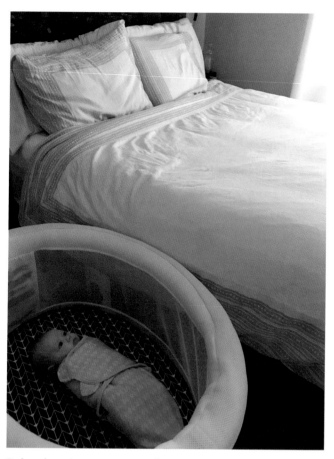

Baby sleeping supine in close proximity to parents' bed but in a separate space

DISTRACTION, ONSET AT 4 MONTHS (BABY, LATER)

Definition

Phase when infant is distracted while nursing, usually at age 4 to 6 months. Infant may have trouble finishing a full feeding and then is hungry and feeds more frequently.

BACKGROUND INFORMATION

- Developmental stage in which an infant is becoming more aware or interested in external stimuli (eg, dog barking, television noise, others talking), which may cause the infant to stop nursing and come off breast

TRIAGE ASSESSMENT QUESTIONS

See Other Protocol

🔘 Low Milk Supply on page 57

See Within 3 Days in Office *(by Appointment)*

🔘 Concern that infant is not getting adequate intake
Reason: milk supply that may be altered by insufficient emptying with distracted infant; may need weight check

Home Care

⚪ Infant pulling off when hearing any noise
⚪ Infant nursing more frequently

HOME CARE ADVICE

❶ **Rest Assured:** This is a developmental phase, but it needs to be addressed because it may result in poor weight gain. Occasionally, a baby does not get full with short feedings and then feeds more frequently, which can be very frustrating for the mother.

❷ **Nurse in Location With Minimal Distraction:** Feed your infant in a quiet, dark room.

❸ **Keep Infant's Attention Toward Breasts:** Stroking your infant's face slowly and gently can be relaxing. Sometimes a necklace with large beads can keep your infant facing inward toward you.

❹ **Minimize Noise:** Avoid talking with others in person or on the phone when nursing.

❺ **Call Back If:** Advice not helping. See within 3 days in office (by appointment).

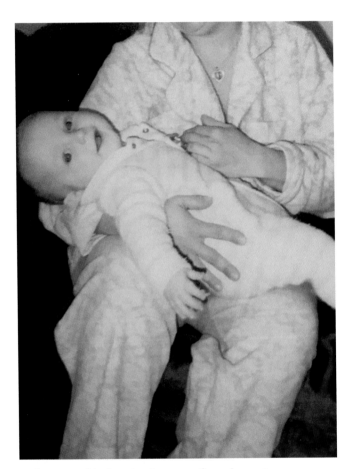

A distracted infant looks away from breast intermittently during a feeding.

EARLY WEIGHT LOSS, BIRTH HOSPITAL OR FIRST WEEK (BABY, EARLY)

Definition

- Early weight loss in the birth hospital of greater than 10% of birth weight may be normal for 5% of vaginal births and 10% of births via cesarean delivery. This is likely due to maternal intake of fluids during the birthing process.
- Close follow-up is warranted, as it may be related to maternal milk production.

TRIAGE ASSESSMENT QUESTIONS

See Other Protocol

- Low Milk Supply on page 57

See Today or Tomorrow in Office *(by Appointment)*

- These mothers are often instructed to do triple feedings (nursing, pumping, and bottle-feeding), and this is difficult to sustain
  Reason: concerns about intake for weight check, as well as pretest and posttest weight evaluation

Home Care

- ○ Baby appears to be nursing and stooling well, and family is reassured by this information

HOME CARE ADVICE

1. **Rest Assured About Weight Loss:** Losing weight early on can be a normal finding. Weight check at the next appointment with the primary care physician can be reassuring. Try to avoid prolonged supplementation or prolonged use of the triple feeding regimen.

2. **Once Weight Is Regained, Return to a More Normal Frequency of Feeds:** Once solved, you need to make sure feedings resume every 2 hours (10–12 feedings in 24 hours).

3. **Keep Awake at the Breast:** Undress to diaper and actively hold your baby's hand or tickle her feet or axilla to keep her awake. Goal is to encourage active suck and swallows and not just shallow flutter feeding.

4. **Skin to Skin:** Having your baby wear only a diaper while laying on your unclothed chest is a good strategy. It can help her get tuned in to feeding.

5. **Call Back If:** Advice not helping or continued concerns. See within 3 days in office (by appointment).

BACKGROUND INFORMATION

- Day 3 to 4 is the most common time for the nadir; 75% of exclusively breastfed newborns regain birth weight by 1 week and 85% by 2 weeks.
- This often sets the family up for undue worry.
- When there is doubt, a referral for a pre– and post–weight check evaluation can turn things around.

EMOTIONAL SYMPTOMS WITH LETDOWN (MOTHER)

Definition

Dysphoric milk ejection reflux (D-MER) is a brief surge of negative emotions (feeling sad, anxious, angry, helpless, hopeless, crying) that immediately precedes letdown and lasts only a few minutes.

TRIAGE ASSESSMENT QUESTIONS

See Other Protocol

- Breast Pain on page 6
- Maternal Postpartum Depression on page 70
- Overactive Letdown/Overabundant Milk Supply on page 86

See Within 3 Days in Office *(by Appointment)*

- Symptoms of sadness that occur at other times not associated with nursing
  Reason: concern for maternal depression; may need referral to mental health professional
- Symptoms that are intolerable
  Reason: evaluation to explore options for medical treatment (eg, bupropion, a dopamine reuptake inhibitor; Rhodiola rosea—golden root [a monoamine oxidase inhibitor that prevents breakdown of dopamine])

Home Care

- ○ Feeling unusually sad or crying before nursing baby
  R/O D-MER
- ○ Feelings of sadness that subside when milk starts flowing
  R/O D-MER
- ○ Large milk supply (Milk may be squirting too fast with letdown.)
  R/O overactive letdown

HOME CARE ADVICE

1. **Rest Assured:** Symptoms of sadness are related to a drop in dopamine with letdown. Simply knowing that D-MER is a described phenomenon should be helpful. It is not postpartum depression because you feel fine at other times. These symptoms often decrease with a baby's age and the number of letdowns.

2. **Take Comfort Measures:** Try relaxation techniques, deep breathing, distraction with music, or aromatherapy.

3. **Connect With Other D-MER Mothers:** May be helpful to network with other mothers through http://d-mer.org.

4. **Consider Overactive Letdown/Overabundant Milk Supply:** May be occurring at the same time. Try feeding in a leaning-back position, and breastfeed on only one side for each feeding.

BACKGROUND INFORMATION

- After milk is released, dysphoria subsides.
- Can occur with nursing, pumping, or letdown without stimulation, such as breast fullness.
- Sensation is associated with a drop in dopamine. This symptom usually self-corrects in 2 to 3 months.
- Typically occurs either with all children or with later children for a mother.

ENGORGEMENT (MOTHER)

Definition
Swelling, fullness, and pain of the larger breast area, usually caused by inadequate drainage of milk from the breast

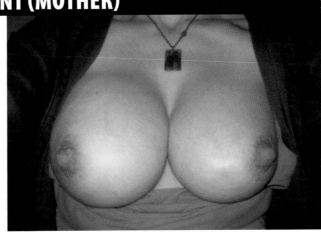

Bilateral breast engorgement

TRIAGE ASSESSMENT QUESTIONS

Go to ED Now (or to Office With PCP Approval)
● Fever, chills, and feel systemically ill
● Engorgement symptoms (pain and hardness to palpation) not improving with home care
Reason: may have mastitis and may need treatment with oral antibiotics or hospitalization for intravenous antibiotics

See Other Protocol
● Breast Pain (plugged duct or mastitis) on page 6
● Sore Nipples on page 93
● Breast Mass on page 4

See Today or Tomorrow in Office (by Appointment)
● Area of redness or tenderness on the skin surface
● Engorgement symptoms (pain and hardness to palpation) not improving with home care
Reason: may have mastitis and may need oral antibiotic treatment or culture if methicillin-resistant Staphylococcus aureus suspected

Home Care
○ Feeling of fullness or even hardness to the breasts on both sides

HOME CARE ADVICE

❶ **Pain Control:** You may take ibuprofen (eg, Advil, Motrin); because of its anti-inflammatory properties, it is the best choice for pain.

❷ **Frequent Feedings:** Breastfeeding is the best way to relieve the discomfort. Nurse approximately every 2 hours (10–12 feedings in 24 hours). If you are too uncomfortable to breastfeed or your baby cannot latch on because of engorged breasts, express milk manually or with a hand or mechanical pump at least every 3 hours (but more frequently if able).

❸ **Warm Comfort:** Taking a warm shower or placing a warm washcloth on the breasts before nursing may help get milk flowing.

❹ **Cold Comfort:** More severe engorgement may require cool compress, such as a gel or an ice pack. Refrigerated, raw, clean cabbage leaves may also provide relief because of their coolness and ability to shape around the breast.

❺ **Reverse-Pressure Softening Technique:** Gentle 2-handed pressure on the breast to push edema away from the areola may help your baby latch better.

❻ **Breast Massage:** In some cultures, vigorous hand massage of both breasts is recommended for engorgement and plugged ducts and can be helpful to get milk moving. However, the massage should not be so vigorous that it causes more discomfort or injures the breast tissue.

❼ **Call Back If:** Advice not helping. See within 3 days in office (by appointment).

BACKGROUND INFORMATION
- Engorgement is most common in the first few weeks postpartum but can occur after a period of separation of mother and baby. May be associated with poor latch.
- Rarely, a mother may have accessory breast tissue with or without an accessory nipple in the axilla or chest, and this becomes evident during this period of early engorgement. Applying direct pressure should suppress milk production in that area.

ENVIRONMENTAL EXPOSURES AND TOXINS (SPECIAL CIRCUMSTANCES)

Definition

Toxins accumulate and are stored in human fatty tissue. Human milk has been used as a biological marker for environmental exposures. It is an easy tissue sample to obtain that represents the adult body's exposure to toxins.

GENERAL CONSIDERATIONS

- The unfortunate backlash is that the public interprets this to mean that human milk is contaminated.
- It is important to realize that studies of laboratory animals and humans show that problems associated with exposure to environmental contaminants are encountered in utero and not during breastfeeding.

Specific Exposures

- **Chlorinated hydrocarbons, such as insecticides (eg, DDT),** are best known and have been studied the longest. DDT is a known carcinogen and affects liver and endocrine systems. Toxins are deposited in body fat and move with the fat into human milk. Extensive summary of studies is available through the National Resources Defense Council (see References on page 111).
- **Polychlorinated biphenyls** are exposures for workers or for mothers who have eaten fish in contaminated waters and have been associated with babies who are small for gestational age when exposure occurs during pregnancy.
- **Dioxins** have been found in mothers with known high-risk exposure, such as those working in dry cleaning, rayon plants, or other chemical industries. Polychlorinated biphenyls and dioxins affect the nervous, endocrine, and reproductive systems of animals and may be carcinogenic.
- **Bisphenol A (BPA)** is used in a variety of consumer products, specifically plastic food and beverage containers, canned foods, and dental sealants. Exposure is ubiquitous in industrialized countries, such as the United States. To avoid excess exposure for breastfeeding babies, BPA-free bottles and pacifiers should be used.

- **Nitrates** can be found in well water. Babies younger than 6 months are particularly susceptible to methemoglobinemia. Levels of 100 mg/L or less do not produce milk with elevated nitrate levels.
- **Heavy metals,** such as lead, mercury, arsenic, and cadmium, can appear in human milk, and levels should be obtained in babies and mothers if an exposure is known.
- **Potassium iodide** should be taken by babies and breastfeeding women if they are contaminated with radioactive iodine and are instructed to do so by government agencies.
- **Formaldehyde** is used as an embalming fluid and can be found in certain laboratories (eg, medical students' anatomy laboratory). Acute exposures are a mucous membrane irritant but are unlikely to enter maternal plasma and affect a nursing baby.
- **Aluminum antiperspirants** are of minimal risk to breastfeeding mothers (animal study showed decreased milk when exposed to high doses of aluminum). If the mother desires, a number of aluminum-free products are available.

TRIAGE ASSESSMENT QUESTIONS

Home Care
○ Concern about a specific environmental toxin and want milk tested

HOME CARE ADVICE

❶ **Call for Testing:** ARUP Laboratories (800/522-2787; www.aruplab.com) can test some toxins in a mother's blood and urine but less so in human milk.

❷ **Rest Assured and Read On**
- Keep breastfeeding because of all the protective benefits.
- According to the Centers for Disease Control and Prevention, "While some women may have detectable levels of chemical agents in their breast milk, no established 'normal' or 'abnormal' levels exist to aide in clinical interpretation. As a result, breast milk is not routinely tested for environmental pollutants."
- For better understanding of this issue, read Steingraber S (see References on page 111).

EXCLUSIVE PUMPING (MILK EXPRESSION)

Definition

- Up to 6% of all breastfeeding mothers pump exclusively as their method of feeding their babies.
- Babies are fed human milk via bottle or cup rather than directly at the breast.
  Note: Pumping is used in this protocol because it is a more common lay term for mechanical expression of human milk.

TRIAGE ASSESSMENT QUESTIONS

See Other Protocol

- No Latch or Inability to Latch on page 82
- Low Milk Supply on page 57
- Sore Nipples on page 93

See Within 3 Days in Office *(by Appointment)*

- Assistance to get baby to latch so mother can direct nurse and stop excessive pumping
  Note: can happen even at 6 months

Home Care

- ○ Pumping only
- ○ Sore breasts and nipples
- ○ Flanges that are rubbing nipples and causing discomfort
- ○ Resentful of the pump/juggling time with baby and a rigorous pump schedule

HOME CARE ADVICE

1. **Encouragement:** The nutritional and health benefits will last a lifetime, but it takes an even greater commitment to maintain milk supply exclusively using a pump. Babies are more efficient at removing milk than any pump.

2. **Pump Use:** Need to use a good-quality double-sided electric pump. Hospital-grade pumps usually need to be rented. Start at a low- to medium-suction setting and increase on the basis of comfort. Stronger suction is not necessarily better and may cause nipple or breast bruising or other trauma.

3. **Nipple Care:** Apply lanolin to nipples before pumping.

4. **Make a Schedule:** Pump for at least 120 minutes in a 24-hour period (translates to 8 times for 15 minutes each) to ensure enough stimulation for a good milk supply. This requires dedication to adhere to a tight schedule every 2 but no longer than 3 hours for the first 2 to 3 months.

5. **Equipment Check:** Make sure that flanges fit well. Nipples should move freely back and forth without rubbing. If rubbing of nipples occurs, larger flanges may be needed (standard is 24 mm, but they come in 21, 27, 30, and 36 mm; glass ones, in 40 mm).

6. **Relaxation:** Deep breathing. Close your eyes and think about your baby. Get comfortable. Cover up the collection bottles with a baby blanket or towel. If you do not focus on every drop as it is expressed, you may be surprised at how much more milk is emptied.

7. **Use of Hands With Pumping:** Use hand massage of breasts while pumping to help with letdown and in obtaining more milk. Can also use warm compresses prior to and during pumping to help with this.

8. **Hands-free Bra:** Helps hold the pump parts so that you can use your hands for another activity while pumping.

9. **Matching Pumping With Desirable Activities:** Plan to read a book or favorite magazine, talk on the phone with a friend or family member, watch a movie or television, or even knit to make pumping more enjoyable.

10. **Skin to Skin While Pumping or at Other Times:** Having the baby nearby or skin to skin (baby wearing only diaper) just before or during pumping can help with milk supply.

BACKGROUND INFORMATION

- Pumping practice usually starts out because of a need to provide milk for a preterm or sleepy baby, latch problems, illness in the mother or baby, separation at birth or later, maternal choice in terms of dislike of breastfeeding at breast, desire for greater freedom, desire for greater control, desire to have others feed the baby, stress or anxiety, or history of sexual abuse.
- This is the choice of a growing number of mothers because they still want their babies to get health benefits of human milk feedings in the first year after birth but do not desire to directly breastfeed or are unable to do so because of return to work or school or other reasons for mother-baby separation.
- Negative feedback is often given to mothers who choose this practice, but sometimes this is the best choice or option for a mother-baby dyad.

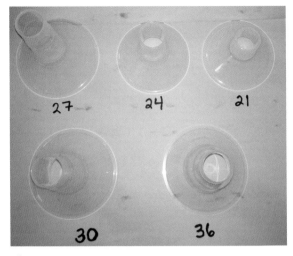

Flanges in various sizes

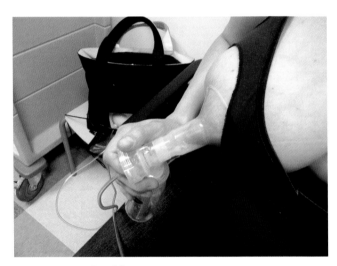

Appropriate fit of flanges

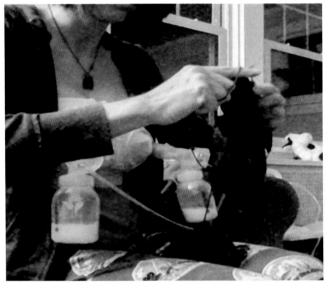

Knitting while pumping

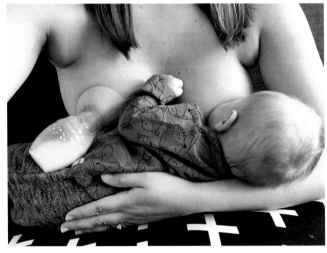

Milk collection system (eg, Milkies) in use on opposite breast while nursing

EXPRESSION OF HUMAN MILK: PUMPING, PARTS AND CLEANING EQUIPMENT, HAND EXPRESSION (ADVICE ONLY) (MILK EXPRESSION)

GENERAL CONSIDERATIONS

- All mothers, even those not returning to work, should have some way to express milk (eg, in case they are delayed at an airport without the baby or at a movie and leaking milk).

When Starting the Milk Expression or Pumping Process

- Best to have a friend or lactation specialist demonstrate pump setup and use. Instructions for assembly can be challenging, especially in the context of sleep deprivation.
- Start with minimal settings and move higher depending on comfort.
- Use lanolin on breasts.
- Nipple should move easily back and forth in the flange without rubbing.

Methods of Expression

Manual (Hand)
One-handed manual pumps are inexpensive and portable and can fit in a large purse. This is a good option for the stay-at-home mother who needs to miss only an occasional feeding because of a night out.

- Manual expression (See Morton J [video] in References on page 111.)
- Hand pump with piston or cylinder
- Hand pump with a squeeze handle or a so-called trigger type (eg, Harmony manual hand pump)

Mechanical
- Battery-operated pumps (2–76 cycles per minute and 8–360 mm Hg pressure) are small and portable but can take a longer time (ie, they are sluggish and should be purchased only if your need is for occasional use).

- Double-sided electric pumps (some have battery pack or cigarette lighter plug-ins).
  - **Large, hospital-grade, dual-action** (eg, Medela Symphony) can be rented, usually monthly, from the delivery hospital or a lactation rental center. These are fast, efficient, and good if you have a late preterm baby for whom the pump will be used for at least a month.
  - **Mid-weight, personal-use, automatic models** (eg, Ameda Purely Yours, Spectra) are comparable to hospital-grade pumps and travel like a briefcase. These are good pumps and best if you are returning to work and will need a long-term option.
  - **Hands-free pumps** (eg, Medela Freestyle) are a good option if you like the idea of doing something else while pumping. Setup is a bit complicated.

Pump Care

- **Cleaning:** Wipe down surface with antibiotic wipes.
- **Sharing of Single User Pumps:** Is not advised. Cross-contamination can happen through the tubing and motor; single user is single user.
- **Parts:** Rinse with hot water after use; may put in dishwasher.
- **Nipple Shields:** Use hot, soapy water; do not put in dishwasher—will melt plastic.
- **Flange Size:** Nipples should move in and out without rubbing against flange.

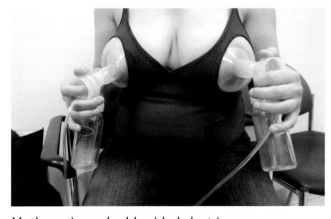

Mother using a double-sided electric pump

The Patient Protection and Affordable Care Act (2010) requires most health insurance plans to cover the cost of a breast pump as part of women's preventive health services. Mothers should contact their insurance provider for specific pump choices.

See Milk Storage and Return to Work/School protocol on page 75.

Options for Breast Pumps From Special Supplemental Nutrition Program for Women, Infants, and Children and Commercial Rental

(Insert local resources here.)

_____

_____

_____

_____

_____

_____

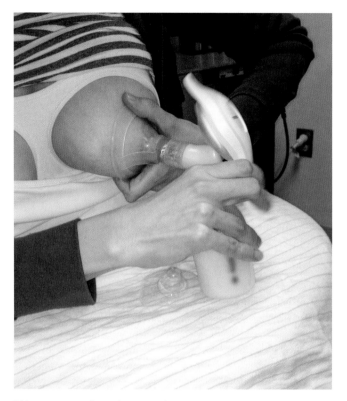

Trigger-type hand pump in use

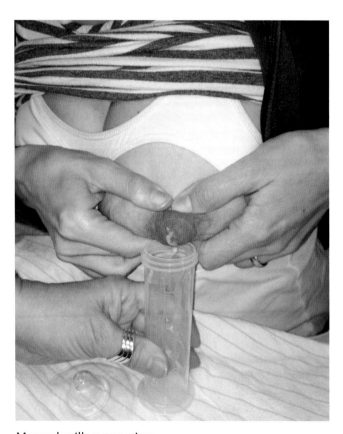

Manual milk expression

FATHERS (ADVICE ONLY) (MOTHER)

GENERAL CONSIDERATIONS

- **Be a Team:** Fathers can be influential supporting cast members when mothers are in the starring role. Fathers are an essential part of the breastfeeding support team.
- **Hold Skin to Skin:** Fathers and families should be encouraged to hold their babies skin to skin after feedings (babies wearing only a diaper lying directly on caregiver's bare chest) because the baby may settle to sleep better, especially if she cannot smell milk (eg, the confusion of "should I eat/ should I sleep" phenomenon for the baby). This is a better task for fathers than bonding while changing diapers!
- **Just Be Nice:** Studies show that being a warm, encouraging presence for the mother is most helpful. This has also been described as valuing the breastfeeding mother and her efforts.
- **Forget About the Chores:** In one study, telling fathers to do the chores, take care of children, do the laundry, etc, actually resulted in shorter breastfeeding duration. Father should focus on mother and baby.
- **Best Thing Is to Help Tired Mother Get a Good Nap:** Fathers should be encouraged to take the baby out of the building so the mother can get carefree sleep at home. Best times to do this are Sunday afternoons or weekend mornings. Father-baby pairs (including older siblings) can go for a walk or to the coffee shop to spend time together, or the father can read the newspaper or work on his laptop while the baby sleeps. This works best if planned in advance so the father can have pumped milk in a bottle just in case, and it should occur shortly after a nursing session. Sleeping through a feeding for mothers can be uncomfortable because of engorgement and is risky in early months because of milk supply.
- **Do Not Criticize the Help:** Mothers (and fathers) should avoid correcting their partners or spouses in terms of baby care, instead catching them doing something right and complimenting them on this.
- **Anticipate Leaking Milk:** A mother's breast can leak and squirt with intimacy, so anticipating this and letting the father know this may happen may be helpful. Some mothers may need a moment to switch

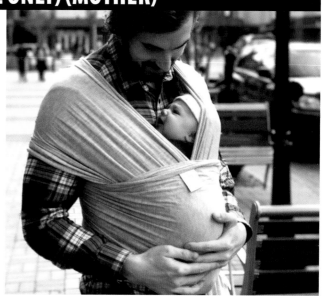

Enjoying an outing with baby in a carrier

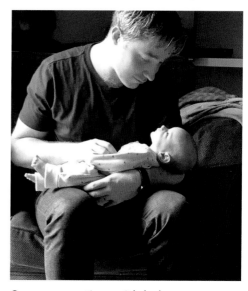

One-on-one time with baby

gears from nursing their baby to having their breasts be part of the intimacy with their spouse or partner.
- **Be Aware of Paternal Depression:** Postpartum adjustment to a newborn can be difficult for fathers too. Expectations around gender in certain cultures can be associated with depression and has been associated with low exclusive breastfeeding. Awareness that about 11% of new fathers may experience depression is important for those working with couples who have a new baby.

FEEDING MORE FREQUENTLY (BABY, EARLY)

Definition
Baby is suddenly feeding more frequently than before (eg, every hour).

TRIAGE ASSESSMENT QUESTIONS

See Other Protocol
- Low Milk Supply on page 57
- Late Preterm Newborn on page 51
- Fussiness, Colic, and Crying in the Breastfed Baby on page 41
- Pacifiers and Slow-Flow Nipples (Advice Only) on page 88

See Within 3 Days in Office *(by Appointment)*
- May be missing a feeding (10–12 times is normal, with 8 as minimum) or be catching up
- Poor latch
- Baby sleepy at the breast
  Reason: concerns about intake for weight check as well as pretest and posttest weight evaluation

Home Care
- ◯ Baby more alert at night or feeding more at night, sleeping more in the daytime
- ◯ Growth spurt: usually at 10 days, 3 weeks, 6 weeks, and 3 months but can vary
- ◯ Cluster-feeding behavior (tanking up at night before a longer stretch of sleep)

HOME CARE ADVICE

❶ **Rest Assured About Growth Spurts or Cluster Feeding:** These behaviors are normal and usually last only 48 hours. Try to avoid supplementation. It is acceptable to feed more frequently during these phases.

❷ **Post-phase Make Certain to Return to a More Normal Frequency of Feeds:** Once solved, you need to make sure feedings resume every 2 hours (10–12 feedings in 24 hours) or to previous routines.

❸ **Day/Night Mix-up:** Need to try to make nighttime quiet and dark and daytime noisy (ie, bring baby into main living area for sleep and, in a few weeks, baby will eventually convert).

❹ **Keep Awake at the Breast:** Undress to diaper and actively hold your baby's hand or tickle her feet or axilla to keep her awake. Goal is to encourage active suck and swallows and not just shallow flutter feeding.

❺ **Roll Side to Side or Change Diaper Between Breasts:** Gently rolling your baby side to side, cradled in both forearms, can be effective. Some wake up with diaper changes.

❻ **Switch Nursing:** Switching sides frequently (every 5 minutes) during a nursing session can keep your baby awake and help with milk supply.

❼ **Try Passing Baby Over to Another Caregiver:** Check if your baby settles with someone besides you after a nursing session; encourage other caregiver and your baby to be skin to skin (ie, baby wearing only diaper on caregiver's bare chest).

❽ **Crying Is Not Always Hunger:** Fussiness is not uncommon at 3 weeks. Try soothing techniques, such as swaddling, swaying, or side-lying position, in caregiver's arms. Some babies have a high suck need, so you may offer a pacifier if it has been at least 90 minutes since the last feeding.
Note: Because pacifiers often lead to missed feeding cues, they should be recommended with caution and only after milk supply is well established (at least 3–4 weeks of age).

❾ **Call Back If:** Advice not helping. See within 3 days in office (by appointment).

BACKGROUND INFORMATION

- Poor latch, inefficient suck, and inadequate milk removal by a baby is most commonly associated with conditions such as large nipple–small mouth mismatch, late preterm newborn, sleepy baby, or a neonatal intensive care unit graduate.
- The baby may have days and nights mixed up, so if he is sleeping more during the day, a feeding may be missed and made up for at night.
- Growth or appetite spurts are typically seen around 10 days, 3 weeks, 6 weeks, and 3 months of age but can vary.
- Cluster or bunch feedings, or tanking up at night, are often seen prior to a longer sleep interval.

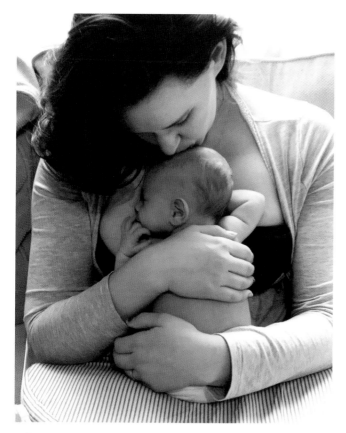

Taking a break from nursing with skin to skin to see if baby is satisfied and will sleep

FEEDING THE BABY WITH CLEFT LIP OR PALATE (SPECIAL CIRCUMSTANCES)

Definition

- Defect, missing tissue, or notch of the lip or palate (roof of mouth) that occurs during fetal development when facial parts are forming.
- These defects can occur separately—20% cleft lip, 30% cleft palate, 50% cleft lip and palate together.
- More often nursing can occur with an isolated cleft lip. Baby can nurse if a seal can form, and at times the breast can even fill the defect.

See Other Protocol

- No Latch or Inability to Latch on page 82
- Exclusive Pumping on page 27

See Today in Office *(by Appointment)*

If these items were not instituted in the hospital before discharge, a more urgent evaluation is indicated.

- Needs access to double-sided pump
  Reason: pumping to establish milk supply and may need plan for long-term mechanical expression, especially if cleft lip and palate
- A special needs feeder or a special cleft palate feeder, an obturator, or both
  Reason: needed if not already introduced at the newborn hospital stay

Home Care

- ○ Cleft lip and baby latched in hospital

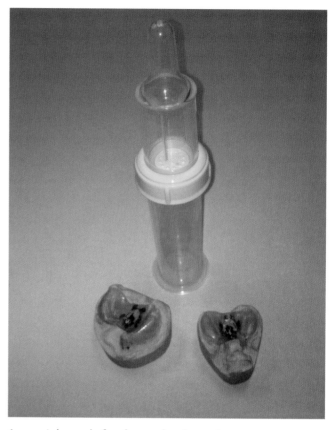

A special needs feeder and palate obturators

HOME CARE ADVICE

❶ Cleft Lip Only and Latched at Birth Hospital: Your baby will need to be followed closely to make sure that adequate milk transfer is occurring. Skin to skin with your baby in only a diaper is a good strategy. It can help babies get tuned in to feeding, with your milk letdown, and with milk supply.

❷ Pumping Plan: Especially in early weeks, you will need to pump every 3 hours regardless if nursing because milk supply may be compromised by ineffective milk transfer.

❸ Cleft Palate: Your baby will likely need an alternative feeding method for optimal growth because of the unlikelihood of achieving negative pressures necessary for adequate milk extraction via direct breastfeeding. Expressed human milk can be fed via a special bottle/nipple, syringe, or gavage tube.

❹ Support: Contact the American Cleft Palate-Craniofacial Association (www.cleftline.org) for information about local support groups for parents of babies with cleft abnormalities.

❺ Call Back If: Advice not helping. See within 3 days in office (by appointment).

BACKGROUND INFORMATION

- Babies with cleft lip and palate should be considered HIGH-RISK and usually encounter significant feeding problems. They also commonly have issues with ear infections, hearing issues, teeth issues, and speech and language delays, making human milk feeding even more important for optimal health, growth, and development.
- Babies with cleft palate cannot compress the breast to create negative intraoral pressures for milk expression, so they usually have a difficult time with nursing. For some babies, use of an obturator (plastic plate for the palate) can help.
- These babies also need careful positioning and support.

- Encouraging mothers to pump and provide human milk for their babies is an important aspect of management. Recent studies indicate that weight gain may be better with breastfeeding versus spoon-feeding for the 6 weeks following surgery.
- Often these babies undergo multiple corrective surgeries in the first few years after birth. This is a long time for mothers to exclusively pump, but many mothers make the commitment, knowing how important their milk is for their baby.
- A recent study indicates that early repair of the cleft lip in the first 2 weeks after birth was associated with higher breastfeeding rates (78%), but in babies with cleft lip and palate breastfeeding rates remained low.

FEEDING THE BABY WITH HYPOTONIA (SPECIAL CIRCUMSTANCES)

Definition
Floppiness or low tone associated with other diagnoses or following a hypoxic-ischemic event after a traumatic birth

TRIAGE ASSESSMENT QUESTIONS

See Other Protocol
● No Latch or Inability to Latch on page 82
● Exclusive Pumping on page 27

See Today in Office (by Appointment)
If these items were not instituted in the hospital before discharge, a more urgent evaluation is indicated.
● Baby who did not latch in the hospital or is latching poorly now
Reason: need for latch and feeding evaluation, possible trial of nipple shield
● Needs access to double-sided pump
Reason: pumping to establish milk supply and may need plan for long-term mechanical expression
● Concern that baby is not gaining appropriate weight
Reason: may need to start supplementation or, if already supplementing, may need to increase caloric density of feeds

Home Care
○ Known diagnosis for floppiness; nursing adequately but may or may not feed better with a bottle

HOME CARE ADVICE

❶ **Skin to Skin:** Having your baby wear only a diaper while laying on your unclothed chest is a good strategy. It can help him get tuned in to feeding.

❷ **Dancer's Hold Position:** Allow your baby's chin to rest on your hand's web space between the thumb and index fingers. The thumb and index fingers can also be used to support your baby's cheeks in this position to enable him to sustain suck longer.

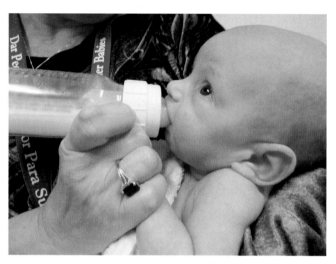
Positioning for feeding a baby with hypotonia

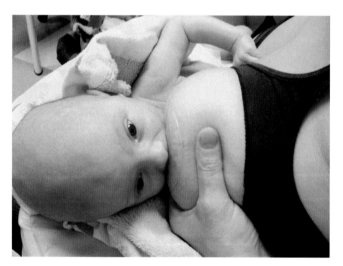
Nursing a baby with hypotonia with a nipple shield

❸ **Use of Pacifiers for Tug-of-war Practice:** Pull on the pacifier but not forcefully enough that it comes out. This has been used in preterm newborns as practice for oral feeding and may be useful with babies with hypotonia.

❹ **Limiting Time at the Breast:** Your baby may need shorter time at the breast if he appears to tire. Follow breastfeeding with supplementation as needed. For some babies, alternating breastfeeding with bottle-feeding can support optimal growth.

❺ **Pumping Schedule:** You will need to pump every 3 hours during the early weeks because your baby's suck may not be strong enough to encourage increased milk production or may not empty the breasts effectively. Your milk supply is established in the first 2 to 3 weeks.

❻ **Call Back If:** Advice not helping. See within 3 days in office (by appointment).

BACKGROUND INFORMATION

- Low tone can be associated with preterm birth, abnormalities of the central or peripheral nervous system, or muscular, endocrine, metabolic, or chromosomal disorders.
- Babies with hypotonia should be considered HIGH-RISK and usually encounter feeding problems.
- They also may need careful positioning and support because of low tone. They often tire easily with feeds.
- Encouraging mothers to pump and provide human milk for their babies is important because of the baby's risk for infections.

FEEDING THE BABY WITH TRISOMY 21 SYNDROME (DOWN SYNDROME) (SPECIAL CIRCUMSTANCES)

Definition

Common genetic birth defect caused by extra genetic material from chromosome 21

TRIAGE ASSESSMENT QUESTIONS

See Other Protocol

- No Latch or Inability to Latch on page 82
- Fortification of Human Milk Recipes (Advice Only) on page 40
- Exclusive Pumping on page 27
- Feeding the Baby With Hypotonia on page 36

See Today in Office (by Appointment)

If these items were not instituted in the hospital before discharge, a more urgent evaluation is indicated.

- Concern that baby is not gaining appropriate weight
  Reason: needs an evaluation, may be related to other abnormalities (eg, heart or respiratory problems); may need to start supplementation or, if already supplementing, may need to increase caloric density of feeds; may need a pulse oximetry evaluation with nursing session
- Baby with associated abnormalities and trisomy 21 syndrome diagnosis (eg, heart or intestinal abnormalities) because it is common that these babies may need increased calories in the form of human milk fortification
- Baby who did not latch in the hospital
  Reason: may benefit from latch and feeding evaluation, possible nipple shield or Supplemental Nursing System, or positioning assistance
- Needs access to double-sided pump
  Reason: pumping to establish milk supply and may need plan for long-term mechanical expression

Home Care

- ○ Baby nursing adequately and may or may not feed better with a bottle

HOME CARE ADVICE

1. **Skin to Skin:** Having your baby wear only a diaper while laying on your unclothed chest is a good strategy. It can help her get tuned in to feeding.

2. **Dancer's Hold Position:** Allow your baby's chin to rest on your hand's web space between the thumb and index fingers. The thumb and index fingers can also be used to support your baby's cheeks in this position to enable her to sustain suck longer.

3. **Use of Pacifiers for Tug-of-war Practice:** Pull on the pacifier but not forcefully enough that it comes out. This has been used in preterm newborns as practice for oral feeding and may be useful with babies with trisomy 21 syndrome.

4. **Limiting Time at Breast:** Your baby may need shorter time at the breast if she appears to tire. Follow breastfeeding with supplementation as needed. For some babies, alternating breastfeeding with bottle-feeding can support optimal growth.

5. **Pumping Schedule:** You will need to pump every 3 hours during the early weeks because your baby's suck may not be strong enough to encourage increased milk production or may not empty the breasts effectively. Your milk supply is established in the first 2 to 3 weeks.

6. **Call Back If:** Advice not helping. See within 3 days in office (by appointment).

Definition

- Babies with trisomy 21 syndrome (Down syndrome) should be considered HIGH-RISK. Usually, half encounter feeding problems because of their small mouths; large, protruding tongues; and low tone.
- They commonly have issues with ear infections, heart defects, intestinal narrowing (microcolon or Hirschsprung disease), pyloric stenosis, and developmental, speech, and language delays.

- Babies with multiple medical conditions have more difficulty with nursing.
- They need careful positioning and support because of low tone, and they often tire easily with feedings.
- If baby has problems breastfeeding, encouraging mother to pump and provide human milk for her baby is important because of the risk of ear and respiratory infections.

FORTIFICATION OF HUMAN MILK RECIPES (ADVICE ONLY) (SPECIAL CIRCUMSTANCES)

GENERAL CONSIDERATIONS

- This protocol should be used to clarify recipes if mother has already been advised by the primary care physician or the neonatal intensive care unit to increase caloric intake of human milk for baby. Normal milk has 20 calories per ounce.
- The Centers for Disease Control and Prevention now recommends mixing the formula with very hot water at 158°F (70°C) to kill any potential *Cronobacter sakazakii* (previously *Enterobacter sakazakii*) prior to adding to the human milk.
- Commercially available human milk fortifiers are generally used for preterm babies and are commonly costlier than donor human milk.

Recipes

- You need to use a measuring spoon used for cooking or baking.
- **For 22-Calorie-per-Ounce Human Milk:** Add ½ **teaspoon** of regular formula powder to 3 ounces of pumped human milk.
- **For 24-Calorie-per-Ounce Human Milk:** Add **1 teaspoon** of regular formula powder to 3 ounces of pumped human milk.

FUSSINESS, COLIC, AND CRYING IN THE BREASTFED BABY (BABY, EARLY)

Definition

- Syndrome in which the young baby has unexplained irritability, apparent discomfort, and crying for a prolonged period, often at a predictable time of day; sometimes referred to as *colic*
- Occurs equally in breastfed and formula-fed babies (about 20%)

TRIAGE ASSESSMENT QUESTIONS

See Other Protocol

- Constipation in the Breastfed Baby on page 18
- Spitting Up (Reflux) on page 96
- Allergy on page 2
- Maternal Ingestion of Foods and Herbs (Advice Only) on page 66
- Overactive Letdown/Overabundant Milk Supply on page 86
- Feeding More Frequently on page 32

Go to Office Now

- Vomiting
  Reason: possible intestinal obstruction
- Swollen scrotum
  Reason: possible testicular torsion, incarcerated hernia
- Difficulty breathing
  Reason: possible pneumonia
- Dehydration suspected: no urine for more than 8 hours and very dry mouth, no tears, sunken soft spot, ill appearing
- Any injury suspected
- Parent who is afraid she might hurt the baby or has spanked or shaken the baby
  Reason: risk for abusive head trauma
- Unsafe environment suspected by triage practitioner
- Baby crying constantly for 2 hours; cannot be comforted after trying for more than 2 hours
  Reason: possible physical or painful cause
- Pain (eg, earache) suspected as cause of crying

See Within 3 Days in Office *(by Appointment)*

- Any symptoms or signs suspicious for allergy (eg, eczema/rash/hives; wheezing; congestion; red, itchy eyes; irritability/colic; vomiting; constipation; diarrhea; family history of allergies)
  Reason: possible allergy to mother's milk
- Any blood or mucus in stools
  Reason: possible allergy
- Extremely fussy most of the time and not just during the late afternoon and evening hours, as with more traditional or usual colic periods
  Reason: possible allergy
  Caution: Conclusions about allergy to dairy should not be made over the telephone because many of these symptoms can occur with other conditions. Dairy allergy occurs in only 2 to 3 of 100 babies. If mother continues to be concerned about possible allergic cause, she can bring diaper/stool sample to an office visit to be tested for blood.

Home Care

- Predictable crying based on time of day or evening
  Reason: if baby is content at other times, probably colic
- Crying related to burping or passing of gas or stool
  Reason: can be normal behavior in young babies if it lasts 10 to 15 minutes
- Baby who has increased gassiness
  Reason: mother who ate gas-producing foods (eg, onions, broccoli, cabbage, beans, turnips, chocolate, apricots, rhubarb, prunes)
- Baby's stools are green and foamy
  Reason: overabundant milk supply or overactive letdown
- Mother taking medications
  Reason: certain medications may have side effects of stimulants in baby; caffeine or energy drink intake

HOME CARE ADVICE

① Rest Assured

- Breastfeeding often gets the blame for any fussiness. Try not to jump to supplementation with formula because changing your baby's diet may add to the problem. Normal crying peaks at 6 weeks of age (at an average of 3 hours in a 24-hour period). Make sure your baby is getting at least 8 feedings in 24 hours. Missing a feeding over a few days can result in a hungry baby who cries.
- Keep your baby on task. If your baby seems hungry, make sure he is awake and actively sucking and swallowing at the breast for all nursing sessions. Holding his hand up in the air or tickling him under the axilla or feet can help.
- Share the care. Your baby may settle better with a non-nursing caregiver after a nursing session. Babies may experience the "should I eat/should I sleep" phenomenon because nursing mothers smell like human milk.
- Temperaments of babies differ. Mothers of breastfed babies may be more in tune with their baby's temperament (and baby's crying is, therefore, more stressful) because of this intimate feeding relationship.

② Hold and Comfort

- Hold your baby skin to skin. Baby, wearing only a diaper, is held on unclothed chest of a parent or caregiver.
- Wear your infant in a sling or another kind of carrier. Safe practices should be emphasized because of the risk of suffocation.
- TICKS pneumonic.
  - **Tight:** Hold in sling so that your baby is tight or snug against you.
  - **In View:** Always keep your baby's face in view of yours. Never cover her face with a blanket.
  - **Close to Kiss:** While your baby is in the sling, always keep her close enough so that you can bend down and kiss her at any time.
  - **Keep Chin Up:** Keep your baby's chin facing up.
    A baby's tucked chin may make it more difficult to breathe.
  - **Support:** Make sure your baby's back feels supported in the sling.

③ Swaddle and Consider the 5 Ss

- Breastfeeding babies need their hands close to their faces for feeding cues, so keep arms tucked up close when swaddling.
- **Consider the 5 Ss,** which are swaddling, side lying, shushing, swinging/swaying, and sucking (see Karp H in References on page 111).
- White noise and car rides are also sometimes helpful for soothing a crying baby.

④ Prevent Gassiness: Consider avoiding or decreasing the amount you consume of common offenders: onions, broccoli, cabbage, beans, turnips, chocolate, apricots, rhubarb, and prunes. Gassiness is usually temporary. If your baby stops having gassiness, consider adding one offender back in at a time over a few days to see if it affects her.

⑤ Reduce Overabundant Milk Supply: If you suspect that you have a large milk supply and associated gassy or foamy, green stools,

- Pump off the foremilk. To help decrease foremilk as well as volume baby may get, at start of feeds (first 5 minutes) pump off the foremilk. Label and save this milk for later; you may need to eventually mix it with other pumped milk.
- Offer only one breast per feed. Best to move to one-sided feedings: allow your baby to finish one side completely; only pump off the undrained side if needed for comfort purposes. This practice allows your baby to get more hindmilk (higher fat, slower gastric emptying) and allows better digestion of lactose from foremilk.

⑥ Review Intake of Caffeine and Energy Drinks: Energy drinks are gaining popularity; examples include Red Bull (80-mg caffeine per 8 ounces) and 5-hour Energy (140 mg per 2 ounces). These should be compared with coffee (108 mg per 8 ounces) when considering risk and advice. Although approximately 3 cups of coffee per day are tolerated in most babies, energy drinks, coffee, and other caffeinated beverages should be used with caution because of caffeine content. It is important to note that caffeine has a longer half-life in babies because it is processed in the liver, and a baby's liver is less mature than a mother's. Babies should be monitored for irritability, insomnia, and increased heart rate.

❼ Contact Fussy Baby Network or Local Fussy Baby Clinic: Call 888/431-BABY (2229). This can be a stressful phase of your baby's development no matter what the reason for the fussiness. Making a telephone call can be helpful, and in some states the family may be offered a home visit or specialty clinic visit.

BACKGROUND INFORMATION

- Neurodevelopmental theory is based on the belief that an overstimulated baby needs to cry as a release.
- Gastrointestinal theory is related to baby reactions to every gas bubble and stool passage with some discomfort and crying. In the breastfed baby, if the mother is eating gas-producing foods, such as cabbage, onions, broccoli, and beans, it can affect the baby.
- Other medical causes for crying should be considered, such as otitis, anal fissure, hair tourniquet, corneal abrasion, torsion, and hernia.
- The breastfed baby may seem unsettled. Smelling the mother can make the baby behave as if he needs to nurse—the "should I sleep/should I eat" phenomenon—so he will settle better with a non-nursing caregiver.
- Foremilk/hindmilk imbalance may be a possibility in mothers with large milk supply. Assistance should be provided to downregulate supply.
- The association of swaddling and sudden infant death syndrome (SIDS) (which was highest in the 6-month-old age range and those who were prone or in side positions) was reported in a recent meta-analysis; therefore, swaddling generates anxiety in families. Reassurance should be provided because swaddling may be helpful in many fussy babies.

GASSINESS IN THE BREASTFED BABY (BABY, EARLY)

Definition

Baby has an increase in frequency of passing gas or appears to have discomfort.

TRIAGE ASSESSMENT QUESTIONS

See Other Protocol

- Maternal Ingestion of Foods and Herbs (Advice Only) on page 66
- Overactive Letdown/Overabundant Milk Supply on page 86
- Spitting Up (Reflux) on page 96
- Allergy on page 2

Home Care

- Baby who has increased gassiness
- Baby's stools are green and foamy
- Overabundant milk or overactive letdown
- Mother who ate gas-producing foods (eg, onions, broccoli, cabbage, beans, turnips, chocolate, apricots, rhubarb, prunes)

HOME CARE ADVICE

❶ **Avoid Gassy Foods:** If present in diet, consider avoiding or decreasing the amount you consume of common offenders—onions, broccoli, cabbage, beans, turnips, chocolate, apricots, rhubarb, and prunes. Gassiness is usually temporary. If your baby stops having gassiness, consider adding one food back in at a time over a few days to see if it affects him.

❷ **Reduce Overabundant Milk Supply:** If you suspect that you have a large milk supply and associated gassy or foamy, green stools,
- Pump off the foremilk. To help decrease foremilk as well as volume your baby may get, at start of feeds (first 5 minutes) pump off the foremilk. Label and save this milk for later; you may need to eventually mix it with other pumped milk.

- Offer only one breast per feeding. Best to move to one-sided feedings: allow your baby to finish one side completely; only pump off the undrained side if needed for comfort purposes. This practice allows your baby to get more hindmilk (higher fat, slower gastric emptying) and allows better digestion of lactose from foremilk.

❸ **Try Warm Bath:** May be soothing for your baby and relax his stomach muscles, thereby helping him pass gas or stool.

❹ **Call Back If:** Advice not helping. See within 3 days in office (by appointment).

BACKGROUND INFORMATION

- In the breastfed baby, increased gassiness may occur if the mother is eating gas-producing foods, especially if in large amounts.
- Foremilk/hindmilk imbalance in mothers with large milk supply; the baby takes in too much foremilk, which can cause a relative lactose overload/intolerance and green, foamy stools.
- Although these foods may result in gassiness, generally restricting maternal diet should be avoided. Exposure to a variety of foods and tastes is normal and may later increase a baby's acceptance of solids.

ITCHING OF THE BREAST/NIPPLE AREA (MOTHER)

Definition

Symptoms of irritation or tickling sensation associated with a persistent need to scratch area of the breast, with or without visible lesions

TRIAGE ASSESSMENT QUESTIONS

See Other Protocol

- Sore Nipples on page 93
- Breast Pain on page 6

See Today or Tomorrow in Office *(by Appointment)*

- Localized redness on skin surface or tenderness of breast
- Pain with palpation
  Reason: if mastitis, may need treatment with oral antibiotics or hospitalization for intravenous antibiotics; pain is a common cause of weaning, so it should be evaluated urgently

See Within 3 Days in Office *(by Appointment)*

- Redness or lesions such as hives/urticaria and exposure to soaps, detergents, perfumes, or creams
  R/O contact dermatitis
- Dry, red, flaky skin and maternal history of eczema
  R/O eczema
- Discrete lesions if redness and serous discharge
  R/O impetigo
- Nipples or areolar area pink, shiny, or flaky
  R/O yeast infection
- Discrete lesions possibly with burrows or tunnels (Infant may have similar lesions.)
  R/O scabies
- Small, raised, hive-like lesions
  R/O spider or other insect bites (eg, mosquito)
- Blister-like lesions with red base
  R/O varicella
- Unilateral nipple that looks as if it has eczema, red and inflamed, associated lump
  R/O Paget disease, inflammatory breast cancer (rare)

HOME CARE ADVICE

❶ Comfort Measures
- Cold pack can be placed on breasts for comfort.
- Oatmeal bath may also be soothing.
- Nonsedating antihistamines may offer relief.
- Hydrocortisone cream, 1%, over the counter as a topical treatment may also be soothing but has not been studied in the nursing infant; any excess should be wiped off before nursing your baby.
- Pramoxine (Sarna lotion) is popular for relief of itching but has not been studied in nursing mothers. Because it is a topical treatment, it is unlikely to affect infants. But, again, any excess is best removed before nursing your baby.

❷ Pain Control: You may take ibuprofen (eg, Advil, Motrin); because of its anti-inflammatory properties, it is the best choice for pain. Acetaminophen (eg, Tylenol) can be added if needed. Both medications are compatible with nursing.

BACKGROUND INFORMATION

Causes

- Most causes are benign, but itching is a challenging and annoying symptom, so mothers may want to be evaluated more urgently. Systemic itching (all over, not isolated to breast area) can be caused by medications or illnesses not covered here.
- **Contact Dermatitis:** Contact with irritants causes burning, cracking, and redness that seems to resolve with removal of the irritant.
- **Eczema:** Usually, mother has some past medical history of dryness or skin irritation.
- **Impetigo:** Superinfection lesions that may have started as skin irritation but now are superinfected with *Staphylococcus*, *Streptococcus*, or both. This will require oral antibiotic treatment.
- ***Candida* (Yeast) Infection:** A mother may also have a pink- or red-tinged nipple area with some peeling, itching, and shininess to the surrounding skin.

- **Mastitis:** At times inflammation of the skin can cause itching. Here also can be pain and redness of the breast, which is often associated with systemic symptoms of fever, chills, and body aches. If pain and tenderness are prolonged, abscess should be considered.

Rare Causes

- **Scabies:** Contagious skin infection caused by the mite *Sarcoptes scabiei*. Usually, other family members have lesions, itching symptoms, or both.
- **Insect Bites:** Such as from spiders or mosquitoes. Exposure may be at night when mother is not aware.
- **Varicella:** Vesicular (tiny blister) lesions on a red base.
- **Paget Disease:** Superficial manifestation of underlying breast malignancy appearing as a small vesicular eruption with persistent soreness, pain, or itching of the nipple or areola.
- **Inflammatory Breast Cancer:** Intense onset of unilateral symptoms such as in Paget disease.

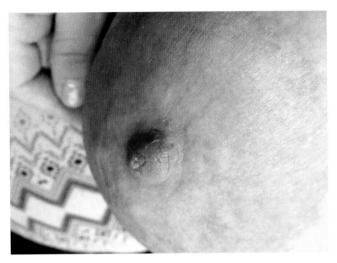

Pink areola and flaky skin suggestive of yeast infection

JAUNDICE, NEWBORN (BABY, EARLY)

Definition

- The skin has turned a yellow color.
- At higher bilirubin levels, the whites of the eyes also turn yellow.
- Included: Home phototherapy questions are also covered.

TRIAGE ASSESSMENT QUESTIONS

Call EMS 911 Now

- Unresponsive and can't be awakened
  R/O: sepsis
- Signs of shock (very weak, limp, not moving, gray skin, etc.)
- Sounds like a life-threatening emergency to the triager

Go to ED Now

- Newborn < 4 weeks with fever 100.4° F (38.0° C) or higher rectally
  R/O: sepsis, UTI

Go to ED Now *(or to Office With PCP Approval)*

- Age 4 - 12 weeks with fever 100.4° F (38.0° C) or higher rectally
  R/O: sepsis, UTI
- Low temperature < 96.8° F (36.0° C) rectally that doesn't respond to warming
  R/O: sepsis
- Newborn < 4 weeks starts to act sick or abnormal in any way (e.g., decrease in activity)
  R/O: sepsis
- Baby sounds very sick or weak to triager
  R/O: sepsis

Go to Office Now

- Feeding poorly (e.g., little interest, poor suck, doesn't finish)
- Signs of dehydration (very dry mouth, sunken fontanelle, no urine in 8 hours)
- Whites of the eyes (sclera) have turned yellow
  Reason: bilirubin level probably over 15

- Skin looks deep yellow or orange or legs are jaundiced
  (Exception: normal skin tone)
  R/O: high bilirubin level
- Jaundice WORSE than when last seen

See Today in Office

- Jaundice spreads to abdomen (belly)
- HIGH-RISK baby for severe jaundice (preterm < 37 weeks or ABO or Rh problem or cephalhematoma or sibling needed bili-lights or Asian race, etc.)
- Began during the first 24 hours of life
  R/O: hemolytic jaundice
- Mother concerned the baby is not getting enough breast milk
  R/O: elevated bilirubin due to poor milk intake
- Good-sized yellow, seedy stools per day are < 3
  R/O: elevated bilirubin due to poor milk intake
  (Exception: breastfed and before 5 days of life)
- Day 2 to 4 of life and no stool in over 24 hours and breastfed
- Wet diapers per day are < 6
  R/O: elevated bilirubin due to poor milk intake
  (Exception: 3 wet diapers/day can be normal before 5 days of life if breastfed)
- Day 2 to 4 of life and no urine in over 8 hours
- Discharged before 48 hours of life and 4 or more days old and hasn't been examined since discharge.
  Reason: AAP recommends recheck
- Caller is concerned about the degree of jaundice
- Caller wants baby seen

See Within 3 Days in Office

- Jaundice begins or reappears after 7 days old
  Reason: not physiologic jaundice
- Stools (BMs) are white, pale yellow, or light gray
  R/O: neonatal hepatitis, biliary atresia
- Jaundice is not gone after 14 days old
  R/O: breast milk jaundice, liver disease, UTI

Home Care

- ○ Mild jaundice of newborn
- ○ Home phototherapy, questions about

HOME CARE ADVICE

Mild Jaundice Treatment

❶ Reassurance and Education:
- Jaundice means the skin has turned yellow.
- Bilirubin is the pigment that turns the skin yellow.
- Bilirubin comes from the normal breakdown of old red blood cells.
- The liver normally gets rid of bilirubin. But at birth, the liver may be immature.
- Half of babies have some jaundice. Usually, it is mild and doesn't need any treatment.
- The first place for jaundice to appear is on the face.
- Jaundice that only involves the face is harmless.
- The level of bilirubin that is harmful is around 20. Reaching a level this high is rare.
- High levels need to be treated with bili-lights. That's why your doctor checks your baby's bilirubin level until it becomes low.

❷ Bottle-feed More Often:
- If bottle-fed, increase the frequency of feedings.
- Try for an interval of every 2 to 3 hours during the day.

❸ Breastfeed More Often:
- If breastfed, increase the frequency of feedings.
- Nurse your baby every 1½ to 2 hours during the day.
- Don't let your baby sleep more than 4 hours at night without a feeding.
- **Goal:** At least 10 feedings every 24 hours.

❹ Infrequent Stools Means Your Baby Needs More Milk:
- Breast milk and formula help carry bilirubin out of the body. Therefore, good feedings are important for bringing down the bilirubin level.
- In the first month, keep track of how many stools are passed daily. The number of stools reflects how much milk your baby is getting.
- If your baby is 5 days or older, he should have at least 3 stools daily. If stooling less than that, it usually means your baby needs more to eat.
- Try to increase the number and amount of feedings per day.

- If you are having any trouble with breastfeeding, consult a lactation expert. Also, schedule a weight check.
- Caution: Stimulating the anus to increase the release of stools is not helpful for reducing the bilirubin level.

❺ Expected Course: Physiologic jaundice peaks on day 4 or 5 and then gradually disappears over 1-2 weeks.

❻ Judging Jaundice:
- Jaundice starts on the face and moves downward. Try to determine where it stops.
- View your baby unclothed in natural light near a window.
- Press on the yellow skin with a finger to remove the normal skin tone.
- Then try to assess if the skin is yellow before the pink color returns.
- Move down the body, doing the same. Try to assess where the yellow color stops.
- Jaundice that only involves the face is harmless.
- As it involves the chest, the level is going up.
- If it involves the whites of the eyes, abdomen, or legs, the bilirubin level needs to be checked.

❼ Call Back If:
- Jaundice becomes worse.
- Eyes, belly, or legs become yellow.
- Feeding poorly or weak suck.
- Baby starts to act sick or abnormal.
- Jaundice not gone by day 14.

Home Phototherapy Questions

❶ Biliblanket—How It Works:
- A biliblanket is a type of phototherapy that can be used at home. It must be prescribed by your baby's doctor. The light emitted from the blanket helps to break down the bilirubin in the skin. The blanket is connected to a machine by a cable. The machine is then plugged into a wall outlet.
- **Safety:** The biliblanket system uses pure light energy so no electricity or heat is generated near your baby. The newborn can't see the light, so no eye patches are necessary.

❷ Biliblanket—How to Put It On:
- The fiber-optic blanket is inserted into a soft cover so it doesn't irritate the baby's skin.

- It emits light from one side only. The bright side is placed directly on the baby's skin and wraps the torso area.
- You can put the baby's clothes over the bibliblanket and swaddle with a regular blanket to keep the newborn warm.

❸ **Bibliblanket—When to Wear It:**
- The blanket should be left on when holding, feeding, or sleeping.
- The only time it's necessary to remove it and turn it off is during bathing.
- In fact, the blanket should be worn as much as possible to be effective.

❹ **Alternate Disposition—Call the Home Health Agency:**
- These babies are usually followed by a home health agency. The home health nurse can assess your baby in the home and provide education. They usually require daily bilirubin tests and weights.
- If you have questions about medical equipment being used in your home, the home health agency may be able to answer them over the phone as well.

❺ **Call Back If:**
- Jaundice becomes worse.
- Feeding poorly or weak suck.
- Your baby starts to act sick or abnormal.

BACKGROUND INFORMATION

Recognizing Jaundice
Sometimes callers aren't certain if the newborn's skin is jaundiced. The color of the sclera is essential in assessing children with darkly pigmented skin. If the sclera are white, the bilirubin level is not worrisome. If the sclera are yellow, the level may be above 15 mg/dL and it needs to be checked.

Bilirubin Level Severity by Parent's Report of Location
- The following rating scale is one factor used for phone assessment in this guideline:
  - **Mild Jaundice:** Face only. Don't need to be seen.
  - **Moderate Jaundice:** Trunk involved (chest and/or abdomen). If the caller thinks the jaundice is worse than when last checked, these newborns need to be brought in for a level.
  - **Severe Jaundice:** Legs involved or entire body surface. Newborns with severe jaundice all need to be referred in for a bilirubin level NOW. The bilirubin level is high if the whites of the eyes (sclera) turn yellow.
- These zones of jaundice probably relate to differences in capillary perfusion and skin temperature.

Bilirubin Measurement
- **Total Serum Bilirubin (TSB):** This is a blood test. It is still considered the "gold standard" and true measurement of the bilirubin. It is done to determine whether babies need phototherapy or not.
- **Transcutaneous Bilirubin (TcB):** This is a noninvasive way to estimate the bilirubin level. A bilirubinometer is placed on the skin and measures the amount of bilirubin present in the extravascular tissue. It is not a substitute for TSB, but it can be used for screening to provide an estimate of the TSB value. If a baby is felt to be at risk for developing clinically significant hyperbilirubinemia, a TSB should be done. The TcB level is not reliable in babies who have received phototherapy.

Causes of Jaundice
- **Physiologic Jaundice (50% of Newborns)**
  - Onset 2 to 3 days of age.
  - Peaks day 4 to 5, then improves.
  - Disappears 1 to 2 weeks of age.
- **Breastfeeding or Malnutrition Jaundice (5 to 10% of Newborns)**
  - Due to inadequate intake of breast milk.
  - Pattern similar to physiologic type.
  - Also causes poor weight gain.
- **Breast Milk Jaundice (10% of Newborns)**
  - Due to substance in breast milk which blocks destruction of bilirubin.
  - Onset 4 to 7 days of age.
  - Lasts 3 to 12 weeks.
  - Not harmful.
- **Rh and ABO Blood Group Incompatibility**
  - Onset during first 24 hours of life.
  - Can reach harmful levels.
- **Liver Disease (Rare)**
  - White or pale stools suggest biliary atresia or other obstructive liver disease as the cause of the jaundice.

Normal Prolonged Jaundice in Breastfed Babies

- At 3 weeks of age, 43% of breastfed newborns have a bilirubin level over 5 mg/dL and 34% were clinically jaundiced.
- At 4 weeks of age, 34% of breastfed newborns have a bilirubin level over 5 mg/dL and 21% were clinically jaundiced.
- These new data should help with reassuring mothers and PCPs that this is normal and usually babies don't require any laboratory tests.
- Source: Maisels, 2014.

Scleral Icterus: A Marker for Significant Bilirubin

- A 2013 study from the University of Pittsburgh Department of Pediatrics (Azzuqa 2013) found that scleral icterus detected by the parent or PCP is a marker for bilirubin levels above 15 mg/dL.
- This finding warrants a bilirubin test.
- None of the newborns with bilirubin levels of 10-15 mg/dL had scleral icterus.

Risk Factors for Severe Jaundice

- Onset within first 24 hours of life.
- Blood type incompatibility (Mother is type O or Rh negative).
- Preterm: Gestational age less than 37 weeks. (Pre-terms are 5 times more likely to have bilirubin levels over 12 than 40-week newborns.)
- Sibling required phototherapy.
- Bruising from birth trauma (e.g., cephalohematoma).
- Breastfeeding, especially if firstborn and feeding not going well. Newborns discharged on Thursday or Friday are at highest risk because they need to be seen on the weekend for a recheck of their jaundice (and sometimes that is overlooked).
- Asian Race: Bilirubin levels over 12 occur in 23% of Asian babies, 12% of whites, and 4% of African Americans.
- Recent phototherapy.
- Caller mentions last bilirubin level was in high-risk zone.

Kernicterus Prevention

- Kernicterus (bilirubin encephalopathy) is the most serious complication of high bilirubin levels.
- Early symptoms are lethargy, hypotonia, poor suck, and high-pitched cry.
- The US kernicterus registry reported 61 cases in term

and near-term healthy newborns in 8 years (Johnson 2002). Currently over 120 cases (2007).

- Bilirubin levels 22-48; 31% idiopathic, 31% G6PD, 10% hematomas.
- **Breastfed:** 59 of 61 (increased risk for dehydration and malnutrition) (97%).
- Sequelae over 90% at 18 months (cerebral palsy, developmental delays, hearing loss).
- See homunculus figure. Zones 4 and 5 are most concerning.
- **Lapses in Follow-up Care:** Only 28% were given an early follow-up appointment within 2-3 days of discharge. (AAP practice parameters 1994 and 2004 recommend any newborn discharged before 48 hours needs a checkup within 2-3 days of discharge for jaundice, feeding behavior, weight, hydration, etc.)
- **Errors in Telephone Care:** Mothers who phoned their doctor's office for jaundice, drowsiness, poor feeding, etc. received repeated reassurance rather than being seen.

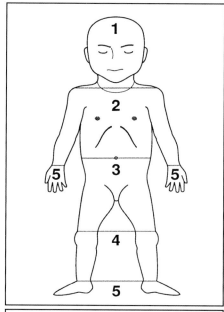

Score	Extent of Jaundice
0	None
1	Face and neck only
2	Chest and back
3	Abdomen below umbilicus to knees
4	Arms and legs below knees
5	Hands and feet

Homunculus used to assign Jaundice Zone Score.

Reproduced, with permission, from Maisels MJ, Clune S, Coleman K. The natural history of jaundice in predominantly breastfed infants. *Pediatrics.* 2014;134(2):e340–e345. © 2014 American Academy of Pediatrics.

LATE PRETERM NEWBORN (BABY, EARLY)

Definition

- Late preterm newborns, defined as 34 to 36⁶/₇ weeks, are particularly at HIGH RISK for nursing issues.
- Early-term newborns 37 to 38⁶/₇ weeks can have difficulties with nursing too.

TRIAGE ASSESSMENT QUESTIONS

See Other Protocol

- 🔴 No Latch or Inability to Latch on page 82
- 🔴 Jaundice, Newborn on page 47
- 🔴 Pacifiers and Slow-Flow Nipples (Advice Only) on page 88

See Today in Office *(by Appointment)*

If these items were not instituted in the hospital before discharge, a more urgent evaluation is indicated.

- 🔴 Newborn who has poor latch and did not feed well in hospital; may or may not have tried nipple shield
  Reason: evaluation for latch, possible nipple shield, and pumping plan for long-term mechanical milk expression
- 🔴 Needs access to double-sided pump
  Reason: pumping to establish milk supply and may need plan for long-term mechanical expression because late preterm newborns often have ineffective suckling and will have trouble with milk transfer
  Note: Nipple shields are made of soft plastic and have holes at the end of the nipple that allow milk to flow through. They are often helpful for newborns who are accustomed to bottle nipple and flow. Again, nipple shields should not be encouraged without lactation supervision, even though they are available over the counter.

Home Care

- ⚪ Baby sleepy on and off at the breast
- ⚪ Newborn nursing adequately and may or may not feed better with a bottle

HOME CARE ADVICE

❶ **Nurse Skin to Skin:** Placing your baby, wearing only a diaper, on your chest is a good strategy. It can help her get tuned in to feeding. It has been shown to help preterm newborns experience more-stable respiratory and heart rates and temperature. Skin-to-skin nursing can help increase milk volume. It will help keep baby awake as well.

❷ **Pump:** You will need to pump for the early weeks until your baby is close to term or is breastfeeding effectively, as evidenced by good weight gain. You may need to pump after feedings as able and offer the expressed milk if your baby is not gaining well.

❸ **Check Slow-Flow Bottle Nipple:** Bottle nipple can be evaluated for slow flow by turning bottle upside down to make sure that no drops of milk come out without squeezing the nipple itself. Fast-flow bottle-feedings may result in newborn preference for bottle and frustration at the breast. Some nipples may be labeled as slow flow but are not. It may require some experimentation to find the nipple that works best for your preterm baby.

❹ **Keep Baby on Task:** If your baby is feeding, trying to keep her awake at the breast is a challenge. Holding her hand up in the air or tickling her under the axilla or feet can help.

❺ **Roll Side to Side or Change Diaper Between Breasts:** Gently rolling your baby side to side cradled in both forearms can be effective. Some babies wake up with diaper changes.

❻ **Switch Nursing:** Switching sides frequently (every 5 minutes) during a nursing session can keep your baby awake and help with milk supply.

❼ **Call Back If:** Advice not helping. See within 3 days in office (by appointment).

BACKGROUND INFORMATION

- Late preterm newborns should be considered HIGH-RISK, and if any symptoms make you suspicious, you should err on the side of prompt evaluation.

- Late preterm newborns may not have a complicated or longer hospital stay, but issues arise when they go home. They should be seen routinely within 1 to 2 days after discharge.
- Right after birth, they commonly have issues with respiratory distress, temperature instability, hypoglycemia, and apnea and, occasionally, with seizures.
- In the first few days after birth, they are at HIGH RISK for jaundice, so bilirubin levels should be evaluated early and followed closely, especially if feeding is not going well.
- Late preterm newborns often have neurologic disorganization with feeding immaturity; suck-swallow-breathe cycle may not be smooth, latch may be poor, suck may be weak, baby may not show feeding cues consistently, and newborn can go from hyperalert to in a very deep sleep, rapidly shutting down.
- They also may need careful positioning and support for their low tone.
- Early-term newborns 37 to 38^6/$_7$ weeks can have difficulties with nursing too.

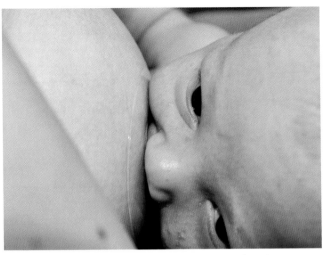

Latch with nipple shield is like training wheels on a bicycle: it keeps baby on task who is getting mostly bottle-feedings.

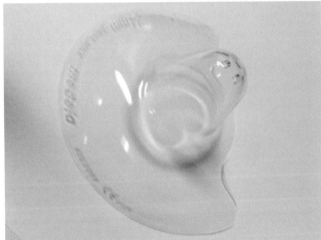

Nipple shield with cutout for nose contact

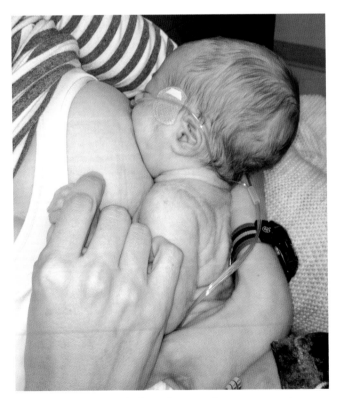

Nursing a preterm baby who requires oxygen via nasal cannula

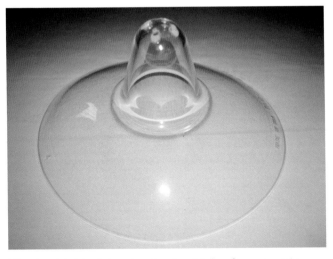

Nipple shield without cutout, which often stays in place better

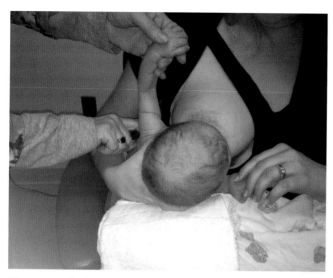

Keeping a baby alert by tickling her under the axilla

LIFESTYLE OR PERSONAL CARE QUESTIONS (ADVICE ONLY) (MOTHER)

GENERAL CONSIDERATIONS

- Most of the concerns presented here are minimal risk. For many mothers, these activities represent returning to a normal lifestyle. This is important for taking some control back into their lives. It is critical to provide encouragement and support in this context if we want to encourage breastfeeding beyond the first few weeks/months after birth. We want mothers to breastfeed exclusively for 6 months and to continue breastfeeding for at least a full year to optimize health benefits for infant and mother.

Hair Color or Permanent Chemicals

- Because minimal amounts are absorbed through the skin, this is considered safe practice.
- Because these inhaled chemicals are lipophilic, acute intoxications potentially could enter maternal plasma and human milk. Hair products should always be used in areas with adequate ventilation.

Nail Salon

- Some polishes contain formaldehyde and toluene. These are regulated by the US Food and Drug Administration. Again, as with hair color, minimal amounts are absorbed through the skin, so nail polish is also considered safe.
- Newer gels and acrylics have not been studied.
- Because these inhaled chemicals can be potentially absorbed into the bloodstream, they should always be used in areas with adequate ventilation.

Tanning Beds

- Care should be taken not to get breasts or nipples burned because of damage to nipples and pain with nursing.
- Vitamins or supplements, sometimes taken to enhance the tanning process, are best avoided.

Exercise

- Exercise is safe in moderation.
- Wear a good supportive bra because some mothers in high-level training situations have had issues with milk supply, and it has been attributed to motion of the breasts and friction to the nipples.

- Time required for training may be difficult to balance in the early newborn period.
- Lactic acid buildup in muscles has been shown to have an effect on human milk taste. If your baby puckers or refuses to nurse, postpone feeding for an hour or replace a feeding with previously pumped milk.
- Care should be taken to avoid dehydration, so adequate hydration is important for maintaining milk supply.

Weight Loss

- Breastfeeding uses 500 extra calories daily from your diet, so by making healthy food choices some women find that return to antepartum weight, or even a lower weight, is enhanced.
- Care should be taken to lose weight slowly because dramatic shifts in weight can affect milk supply.
- Supplements and weight loss pills are not well studied in nursing mothers and are best avoided.

Overweight/Obesity

- Mothers with prepregnancy body mass index greater than or equal to 30 or with previous Lap-Band procedures for weight control (even with now normal weight) are at risk for low milk supply.
- Cause is not clear, but it may be a combination of hormonal influences on breast tissue (hyperinsulinemia), psychological issues (body image), and mechanics for latch. Evaluation should be sought early in the postpartum period.

Acupuncture

- Used for increasing milk supply, but evidence is mixed on effect on prolactin.

Tattoos

- Tattoo ink molecules are too large to pass into human milk.
- Opinion favors waiting to get a new tattoo until the mother is not nursing because of the risk of tetanus, hepatitis B, hepatitis C, and HIV infections with use of tainted needles.

Botox Injections

- Botox is a large molecule that should not pass into human milk, and it tends to remain in the muscle when injected.
  Precaution: Do not breastfeed for 4 to 6 hours postinjection.

Nipple Piercing

- Generally thought to not impede breastfeeding; case reports of nipple piercing have shown that nipple trauma and scarring can cause blocked ducts.
- It is recommended that the ring stay in place for 6 to 10 months minimum after initial piercing, but the hardware should be removed to ensure good latch and avoid choking your baby.

Energy Drinks

- Energy drinks are gaining popularity; examples include Red Bull (80 mg of caffeine per 8 ounces) and 5-hour Energy (140 mg per 2 ounces). These should be compared with coffee (108 mg per 8 ounces) when considering risk and advice.
- Although drinking approximately 3 cups of coffee per day is tolerated in most babies, energy drinks, coffee, and other caffeinated beverages should be used with caution because of the caffeine content. It is important to note that caffeine has a longer half-life in babies because it is processed in the liver, and a baby's liver is less mature than a mother's. Babies should be watched for irritability, insomnia, and increased heart rate.

Placental Encapsulation

- Some mothers have their placenta made into dehydrated capsules to ingest postpartum. There was one case of late onset group B *Streptococcus* contracted to the baby through this practice.

Breastfeeding or Use of Human Milk During Painful Procedures for Infants

- Use of sucrose is common for painful procedures such as circumcision. Nursing during immunizations or providing human milk during painful procedures, such as eye examinations, has been associated with reduced crying and composite pain scores in babies.

Travel

With Baby

- Traveling with a breastfeeding baby can be easier because extra supplies and formula preparation are not needed. Using a sling or carrier to keep your baby close to your body can protect him from environmental exposures and physical contact from well-meaning strangers and germ-carrying older children.

Without Baby

- Planned travel away from a baby should not be a reason to not breastfeed. You should be able to express milk for 2 to 3 days easily with a double-sided electric pump.
- Battery packs offer flexibility and less stress in finding an outlet for plugging in.
- For a longer business trip (≥1 week), try to arrange for a family member or a hired caregiver to travel with you so that your baby can feed at times when you are not working. This is the ideal for maintaining milk supply.
- If it is not possible to bring your baby along, planning a few days off after you return to reunite with him and nurse more frequently is also desirable for all!
- Declare more than 3 ounces of human milk to security officers at security checkpoints; separate it from other liquids, gels, and aerosols in quart-sized, resealable storage bags. These items may be subject to additional screening (eg, you may be asked to open a container), but no one will be asked to taste human milk.
- Use similar procedure at customs.
- A breast pump is considered a personal item and can be carried on and stored in the overhead bin like a laptop computer.

See Other Protocol

- Alcohol Use on page 1
- Marijuana Use on page 61
- Milk Storage and Return to Work/School on page 75
- Expression of Human Milk: Pumping, Parts and Cleaning Equipment, Hand Expression (Advice Only) on page 29

LONG-TERM BREASTFEEDING (ADVICE ONLY) (BABY, LATER)

TRIAGE ASSESSMENT QUESTIONS

See Other Protocol
- Nursing With Pregnancy on page 85
- Tandem Nursing on page 100

GENERAL CONSIDERATIONS

Adding Solids to Milk-Only Diet
- Complementary foods are not needed until about 6 months of age and should not be introduced before 4 months of age.
- Iron and zinc stores are most crucial, so you may start first complementary feedings at 6 months with rice cereal or bananas, but you should move quickly to ground-up meats.
- Myths exist around rice cereal assisting with sleep (alone or when mixed in with human milk), but no evidence suggests that this makes a difference.

Adding Carton Milk After 1 Year
- If you are nursing your toddler 2 to 3 times in 24 hours, it is not necessary to offer supplemental bovine milk when species-specific human milk is available!
- Other liquids can include water or less than 4 ounces of 100% juice per day. Offer liquids in a sippy cup; no bottle is needed.

Immune System Protection and Other Effects of Continued Breastfeeding After 1 Year
- Immune system protection continues and is dose dependent.
- No upper age limit for nursing exists, according to the 2012 American Academy of Pediatrics "Breast-feeding and the Use of Human Milk" policy state-ment, as well as to World Health Organization/United Nations Children's Fund guidelines.
- Nursing can go on for a long time without you needing to pump (with 2-times-a-day nursing).
- It may be difficult to express milk with a pump when your child is at this older age.

- Once you get pregnant again, you may experience breast or nipple pain, and your child may notice a change in taste or amount of milk. As you approach the delivery date, your milk resumes its colostral phase of production to prepare for your new baby.
- Occasionally, some toddlers/children may nurse frequently (sometimes called "grazing") and will not have an appetite for a varied diet of solid foods. If growth is faltering, do not offer fluid 2 hours before meals to maximize the opportunity for a good appetite for meals.

LOW MILK SUPPLY (MOTHER)

Definition

- Perception that human milk coming from the mother's breasts is not enough to feed or satisfy her baby. This is an important concern to address early on because it is the main reason (35%) for early cessation.
- Mothers may feel insecure about their milk—yellow at first (colostrum) and then, once milk is in, a white, watery substance coming from the breasts.
- The belief that all a baby needs is coming from the mother's own breasts (that may have never been used for this purpose before) is a stretch for most mothers.

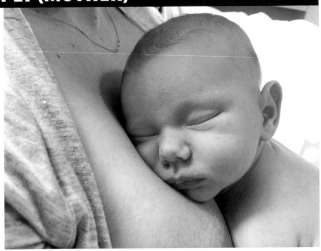

Skin to skin with baby can help with supply.

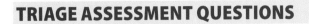

TRIAGE ASSESSMENT QUESTIONS

See Other Protocol

- Feeding More Frequently on page 32
- Fussiness, Colic, and Crying in the Breastfed Baby on page 41
- Contraception, Lactation Amenorrhea Method (Advice Only) on page 19
- Maternal Medications (Advice Only) on page 67
- Breastfeeding in the First Few Weeks: Simplify Your Life (Advice Only) on page 10
- Low Milk Supply in Older Baby >6 Months (± decrease in pumping volumes) on page 60

Questions About Pregnancy

- Fertility issues and possible polycystic ovary syndrome
- Medical problems in pregnancy
  Reason: complications can cause delay in lactogenesis
- Gestational diabetes (4% of pregnancies)
  Reason: hyperinsulinemia can be associated with low milk supply
- Breast surgeries, such as reductions or implants
  Reason: scar tissue or nerves may be affected
- Any thyroid problem
  Reason: can interfere with hormones needed for lactation

- Inadequate weight gain (ie, fewer than 20 pounds)
  Reason: too little weight gained is associated with lower milk supply
- Prepregnancy overweight
  Reason: obesity is associated with lower milk supply
- No breast changes during pregnancy (larger size, increased veins, tenderness)
  Reason: suspect glandular insufficiency

Questions About Hospital Stay

- Difficult or cesarean delivery
  Reason: complications can cause delay in lactogenesis
- Significant blood loss
  Reason: suspect Sheehan syndrome with associated hypopituitarism
- No or poor latch in hospital
  Reason: inadequate stimulation early on can cause a decrease in milk supply
- Medications such as oral contraceptives or pseudoephedrine
  Reason: some medications and contraceptives can affect milk supply
- Baby who has any medical issues
  Reason: any separation or illness can affect latch and early feeding
  Reason: see primary care physician or lactation specialist because mother and baby need evaluation for milk supply; weight check and a pretest and posttest weight visit can be helpful parts of the assessment

Home Care

○ Baby more alert at night or feeding more at night, sleeping more in daytime

○ **Growth Spurt:** usually at 10 days, 3 weeks, 6 weeks, and 3 months, but times can vary

○ Cluster-feeding behavior (tanking up at night before a longer stretch of sleep)

○ First 2 weeks after birth and weight loss of less than 10% of birth weight

○ After 2 weeks, recent weight check that reveals adequate weight gain

○ Normal stooling pattern for age

HOME CARE ADVICE

❶ Rest Assured: Insecurity about milk supply is common. The belief that all a baby needs is coming from the mother's own breasts is a stretch for most mothers. Most mothers can make sufficient milk to feed their babies. Fewer than 5% of mothers have insufficient breast tissue to make adequate milk. Getting in a nap, drinking to satisfy thirst, and decreasing stress (increased cortisol levels can inhibit prolactin) all are helpful. (For more suggestions, see Breastfeeding in the First Few Weeks: Simplify Your Life [Advice Only] on page 10.)

❷ Review Latch: Relax and talk to your baby. Try tickling your baby's upper lip with the nipple, and wait for her mouth to open wide. Then latch her on with the nipple aiming to roof of the mouth.

❸ No Magic Bullet

• Although some evidence shows that fenugreek, nonalcoholic malt, and metoclopramide may increase milk supply, there is, unfortunately, no magic bullet.

• Frequent milk removal with your baby at the breast or expression with a pump is the most effective way to increase or maintain milk supply.

• Mothers are increasingly being placed on or seeking out through Internet pharmacy means the medication domperidone. Domperidone is a potent dopamine D_2-receptor antagonist, with a dosage range from 30 to 60 mg, and stimulates the release of prolactin. It has been shown to be only mildly effective. Because adverse effects of drug-induced long QT syndrome (abnormal heart rhythm and sudden death) occurred

mostly in women, it is not approved for use in the United States by the US Food and Drug Administration.

• Many cultures recommend consumption of foods high in protein, such as fish soup or atole. These customs have been used throughout history and may help milk supply as an adjunct but should not replace milk removal as the primary approach to low milk.

• **Tea:** Historically, some cultures have used teas as galactagogues. Ixbut or euphorbia has been used by the Mayans for centuries. Green papaya or papaya enzyme is popular in Asian cultures. Mother's Milk tea with blessed thistle is also recommended; however, these have not been formally studied.

❹ Keep Track of Feedings: Make sure you are feeding every 1½ to 2 hours (10–12 feedings in 24 hours). Keep a pad of paper handy and make hash marks to help keep track of feeding; use an app or a spreadsheet to document. Missed feedings can affect milk supply. Pay attention to your baby's early feeding cues, such as bringing the hands to the face; do not allow him to get to the hungry/ grumpy crying stage.

❺ Keep Baby on Task: Trying to keep your baby awake at the breast can be a challenge. Holding his hand up in the air or tickling him under the axilla or feet can help.

❻ Roll Side to Side or Change Diaper Between Breasts: Gently rolling your baby side to side, cradled in both forearms, can be effective. Some babies wake up with diaper changes.

❼ Switch Nursing: Switching sides frequently (every 5 minutes) during a nursing session can keep your baby awake and help with milk supply.

❽ Normalize Crying: Crying is a normal baby behavior, and it is not always caused by hunger. Fussiness is not uncommon in the first months. Try soothing techniques, such as swaddling, swaying, and side lying, to calm your baby prior to feeding. Check if she settles with someone besides you after a nursing session, especially skin to skin.

❾ Call Back If: Advice not helping or continued concerns. Better to come in for a weight check office visit (by appointment).

Callback: Assessment of Milk Volume

- Ask mother to express milk manually or with an electric pump. Call her back in 30 minutes and see how many milliliters she has pumped. In early days, reference range volumes include 15 mL or less of colostrum; once milk is in (days 3–5), 1 to 2 ounces is normative. A newborn stomach is the size of a chicken egg.

BACKGROUND INFORMATION

- Early weight loss in the birth hospital of greater than 10% may be normal for 5% of vaginal births and 10% of births via cesarean delivery. This is likely due to maternal intake of fluids during the birthing process and often sets the family up for undue worry. Day 3 or 4 is the most common time for the nadir; 75% of exclusively breastfed newborns regain birth weight by 1 week and 85% by 2 weeks.
- Less than 5% of mothers have primary glandular insufficiency as cause of inability to produce milk.
- Poor latch and inadequate milk removal by the baby.
- Constantly feeding "every hour" because the baby is sleepy or ineffective feedings at breast (caused by congenital abnormality or hypotonia).
- Perceived low milk can occur with a baby's cluster-feeding behavior because of normal growth or appetite spurts.
- Occasionally, low milk supply can be hormonally related to obesity, hypothyroidism, polycystic ovary disease, or infertility.
- Any breast surgery (eg, reduction, augmentation, removal of mass or cancer).
- Surprisingly, nutritional intake of the mother is not as important because milk composition is unaffected, even in malnourished mothers in underdeveloped countries.
- Complications with vaginal or cesarean delivery (eg, hypertension, blood loss, retained placenta) can delay milk coming in as well as diminish milk supply.
- Hormonal contraceptives and medications such as pseudoephedrine.

Checklist for Risks of Low Milk (and Should Be Getting Close Follow-up for Breastfeeding Support and Evaluation of Milk Transfer)

✓ Late preterm or small for gestational age
✓ Neonatal intensive care unit stay because of preterm birth or other cause
✓ No latch in birth hospital
✓ Birth by cesarean delivery or difficult delivery
✓ Early cessation with previous baby
✓ Multiples
✓ Mothers with breast biopsy or surgery
✓ Mothers who are supplementing more than 2 times in 24 hours

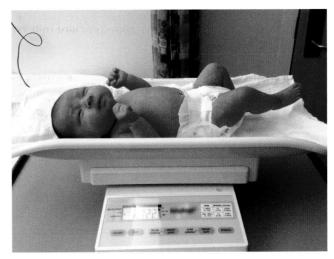

Baby on special scale for pre- and post-weight measurement (ie, measures down to the gram)

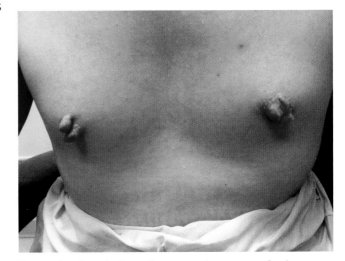

Example of variation of maternal anatomy for low milk supply

LOW MILK SUPPLY IN OLDER BABY >6 MONTHS (MOTHER)

Definition

Mothers who have been nursing and pumping for 6 months or more now experience a drop in milk supply.

TRIAGE ASSESSMENT QUESTIONS

See Other Protocol

- Feeding More Frequently on page 32
- Contraception, Lactation Amenorrhea Method (Advice Only) on page 19
- Maternal Medications (Advice Only) on page 67

Home Care

- Feedings start to take less time; baby is more efficient at removing milk from mother's breast
- Starting solids begins to decrease baby's appetite
- Starting gradually may have less of an effect on appetite
- May have a satisfied baby at breast because he gets enough if directly nursing, but pumping results in lower volumes
- Return of menstruation or ovulation can result in a temporary drop in milk supply
- Hormonal changes due to contraception or pregnancy

HOME CARE ADVICE

❶ Reassurance: This is a common concern with older babies. The amount of milk you pump is not a measure of the milk supply available to your baby at the breast. Try not to panic and offer unnecessary formula supplementation.

❷ Communication With Child Care: Baby may be getting large volumes during the day when not with mother and not stimulating breasts enough during together times. If your baby is in child care, it may be time to limit large volumes in the bottle (eg, 4 ounces may be a sufficient volume at this age). Offer your baby a sippy cup with water at solid meals.

❸ Mother Self-care: Stress, inadequate sleep, restrictive diet, not drinking enough fluid, illness, and mastitis can have small additional effects on milk supply with an older infant.

BACKGROUND INFORMATION

- This is a common concern for telephone calls and blogs, and it usually is only temporary and easily explained by the information included herein.

MARIJUANA USE (MOTHER)

Definition

- Marijuana (tetrahydrocannabinol [THC]) transfers readily into human milk, and it is stored in fat.
- Secondhand smoke from marijuana has many of the same cancer-causing chemicals as smoke from tobacco.
- Breastfeeding mothers should not use marijuana.

TRIAGE ASSESSMENT QUESTIONS

Go to ED Now

⬤ Symptoms of irritability or sedation in the baby of a mother who has smoked or ingested marijuana recently
Reason: evaluation of baby for marijuana intoxication

BACKGROUND INFORMATION

- Limited research is available on breastfeeding and marijuana use, including on amount of THC in human milk, length of time THC remains in human milk after exposure, and effects on infants. Because of concerns for the developing brain in infants, mothers should abstain from using marijuana while breastfeeding.
- Although some institutions have been using negative results from a urine toxicology screening after exposure as an end point to resume breastfeeding, it has not been studied and is not recommended.
- Paternal use of marijuana has been associated with sudden infant death syndrome.
- Resources to help mothers stop using marijuana include 800/CHILDREN (English) or 866/LASFAMILIAS (Spanish).

MATERNAL ANESTHESIA/ANALGESIA (ADVICE ONLY) (MOTHER)

Definition

Breastfeeding after pharmacologic pain control given to breastfeeding mother with painful procedures or surgery

GENERAL CONSIDERATIONS

Anesthesia Medication

- Regional anesthesia (epidural or intrathecal/spinal) is preferred over general anesthesia because less anesthetic gets into human milk.
- Anesthetic gases are cleared quickly from your systemic circulation. Most anesthetics enter the plasma only briefly, so their presence in human milk is low and, therefore, safe.
- Separation of you and your baby should be minimized and breastfeeding initiated as soon as feasible unless your baby is preterm or subject to apnea.
- You may breastfeed postoperatively as soon as you are alert enough to hold your baby; your alertness means that the medications have left your blood and are now in adipose and muscle tissue. A single pumping and discarding following surgery will eliminate any questionable risk.
- It is best to find out in advance what medications will be used. Most mothers are not aware of what medications will be used even for such things as dental procedures. Although shorter-acting agents, such as fentanyl and midazolam, may be preferred, single doses of diazepam are also unlikely to affect the breastfeeding baby. For more extensive information on specific agents, please see Academy of Breastfeeding Medicine Protocol #15, revised 2017 (www.bfmed.org).

Oral Pain Medications for Postoperative Pain Management

- **Ibuprofen (eg, Advil, Motrin), ketorolac, celecoxib, and naproxen, which all have low milk transfer levels, and acetaminophen (eg, Tylenol)** are medications that can be used safely for pain relief. One possible case report exists of a breastfed 7-day-old who had gastrointestinal bleeding whose mother was taking naproxen. Shorter-acting nonsteroidal anti-inflammatory drugs (commonly referred to as NSAIDs) are preferred in the preterm or term newborn.
- **Hydrocodone:** Has been used worldwide by breastfeeding mothers, and less than 4% reaches the baby. Higher doses (30 mg) and frequent dosing can lead to sedation. It should be used with caution because some mothers are rapid metabolizers, and cases have been reported of apnea and death in babies from toxic levels of codeine metabolite.
- **Oxycodone (Percocet):** Once your milk comes in, oral oxycodone (and combinations) can be used, with a maximum dosage of 30 mg daily, as well as supplementing analgesia with a nonnarcotic analgesic if necessary. Maximum oxycodone dosage is 30 mg daily. Again, less than 4% gets into human milk, but prolonged and frequent administration may lead to neonatal sedation.
- **Tramadol:** Previously considered a safe choice; recently, the US Food and Drug Administration recommended against its use in breastfeeding women.

See Other Protocol

- Maternal Medications (Advice Only) on page 67

MATERNAL CONTRAINDICATIONS/CAUSES FOR CONCERN WITH BREASTFEEDING (ADVICE ONLY) (MOTHER)

CONTRAINDICATIONS

Medications
- Chemotherapeutic/antineoplastic agents
- Amiodarone
- Chloramphenicol
- Ergotamine
- Gold salts
- Phenindione
- Radioactive pharmaceuticals
- Retinoids
- Tetracyclines (chronic for >3 weeks)
- Certain psychotropic medications

Infections
- HIV infection.
- Active herpes or varicella lesions of the nipple or areola (baby can nurse on unaffected side).
- Active tuberculosis until mother is treated and considered to be no longer contagious with her respiratory droplets.
- Varicella (close to delivery), but baby can nurse with vaccine on board.
- Hepatitis C with active bleeding of nipples.
- Ebola disease. When safe alternatives to breastfeeding and infant care exist, mothers with probable or confirmed Ebola disease should not have close contact with their infants (including breastfeeding). It is not clear when it is safe to resume breastfeeding after a mother's recovery, unless her milk can be shown to be Ebola disease–free by laboratory testing.
- Zika virus infection. Case reports indicate possible transmission through human milk.

Illicit Drug Use
See Substances of Abuse (Illicit Drugs) protocol on page 99.

CAUSES FOR CONCERN
- Situations that, until clarified or confirmed, mean mother should continue pumping her milk but supplement with banked pasteurized donor human milk or formula in the interim (until her primary care physician determines safety of maternal condition for lactation and feeding).
- **Medications:** Lithium (requires close follow-up of levels and symptoms in mother and baby), pseudo-ephedrine (can affect milk supply).
- **Radiologic Procedures:** Use of radioactive dyes was previously thought to be a contraindication, but less than 1% of the contrast medium is found in human milk ingested by the baby and absorbed by the intestinal tract. This applies to iodinated x-ray contrast media as well as gadolinium-based contrast agents. Some sources say that "if mother remains concerned, she can pump for 24 hours and discard the expressed milk," but this is not necessary.

NOT OF CONCERN
- Maternal hepatitis B is compatible with breastfeeding as long as baby receives hepatitis B immunoglobulin and vaccine.

See Other Protocol
- Maternal Illnesses (Advice Only) on page 64
- Exclusive Pumping on page 27
- Maternal Smoking, Vaping, and Cessation Strategies on page 73
- Substances of Abuse (Illicit Drugs) on page 99
- Alcohol Use on page 1

HOME CARE ADVICE

Pumping Until Evaluation Is Best: It is safest for you to use a pump every 3 hours and store your milk until referral can be made for evaluation. Supplement with donor human milk or formula until evaluation occurs.

MATERNAL ILLNESSES (ADVICE ONLY) (MOTHER)

Definition

Mother is acutely sick or has a chronic condition that affects her ability to nurse or necessitates careful medication choices. Nursing should continue whenever possible because of almost instantaneous transfer of antibodies.

TRIAGE ASSESSMENT QUESTIONS

See Other Protocol

- Maternal Postpartum Depression on page 70
- Maternal Contraindications/Causes for Concern With Breastfeeding (Advice Only) on page 63
- Breast Pain (for mastitis) on page 6
- Sore Nipples (for Raynaud disease of the nipple/vasospasm) on page 93
- Maternal Medications (Advice Only) on page 67

GENERAL CONSIDERATIONS

- Mothers should continue breastfeeding when ill or febrile, nurse more frequently, and practice frequent handwashing.
- If mother is so ill that she cannot nurse, she should be encouraged to pump to maintain milk supply and have another caregiver feed her baby with expressed human milk.
- Mothers who receive transfusions for postpartum hemorrhage are 10% less likely to be breastfeeding at discharge and may need close follow-up.
- Underlying chronic illness can interfere with a mother's well-being and needs to be addressed in the context of medication and management decisions to ensure that breastfeeding can continue safely.
- LactMed (http://toxnet.nlm.nih.gov/newtoxnet/lactmed.htm), Infant Risk Center (www.infantrisk.com; 806/352-2519), and Motherisk (www.motherisk.org; 877/439-2744) are all useful sites for any medication and breastfeeding compatibility questions. *Note: Common illnesses are addressed here, but for more extensive information on chronic illness and infectious transmission, please refer to References on page 111.*

Specific Illnesses

- **Common Cold:** Popular remedies include use of vitamin C; dosage of 120-mg vitamin C is safe in lactation, but usually most mothers get enough from their diets and do not require supplementation. Zinc has been shown to stop rhinovirus from replicating, and taking 25 to 50 mg is considered safe in lactation. Use of pseudoephedrine in over-the-counter cold medications should be avoided, as it can affect milk supply.
- **Influenza:** Reports of viremia are rare, and antiviral medication or prophylaxis is safe. During the H1N1 scare, recommended precautions included handwashing and, if sneezing or coughing, wearing a face mask or covering the mouth and nose with a tissue.
- **Urinary Tract Infection:** For uncomplicated urinary tract infection, ciprofloxacin, nitrofurantoin, and ofloxacin are safe choices for outpatient oral treatment. Trimethoprim-sulfamethoxazole (Bactrim) should not be used as first-line treatment when nursing preterm newborns or if the baby is younger than 1 month because of issues with glucose-6-phosphate dehydrogenase and hyperbilirubinemia.
- **Asthma:** Management should continue the same as before pregnancy because all medications are generally safe for breastfed babies. Less than 10% of inhaled medications gets absorbed into plasma (applies to long-acting beta-agonists, mast-cell stabilizers, and inhaled steroids), and they are considered safe for baby.
- **Allergic Rhinitis:** Nonsedating antihistamines, nasal steroids, and topical eye preparations are all safe.
- **Migraine Headache:** Ibuprofen (eg, Advil, Motrin) and acetaminophen (eg, Tylenol) are the safest choices but are not always adequate treatment for migraines. Triptans are usually the first-line treatment and are considered safe. Ergot alkaloids should be avoided. Peppermint oil rubbed on temples has been used but can suppress lactation.

- **Attention-Deficit/Hyperactivity Disorder:** Limited evidence indicates that medications such as methylphenidate have low levels in milk. Neurologic effects on the baby have not been well studied. Because mothers with this disorder are at risk for psychosocial and parenting difficulties, discussions with their primary care physician are warranted.

- **Hypertension:** Primary hypertension of unknown etiology should be treated with salt restriction. Best medication choices include methyldopa, labetalol, and hydralazine. For other etiologies, medication is guided by underlying pathology. Mothers who have hypertension prepregnancy are at risk for pre-eclampsia and subsequent hypertension.

- **Seizures:** Epilepsy is treated with many different medications; therefore, close consultation with a neurologist is best for the nursing mother. Phenytoin, carbamazepine, valproic acid, and levetiracetam appear to be safe choices. Gabapentin and lamotrigine should be used with caution. These medications can cause drowsiness in infants and may affect milk transfer at the breast. If there are any concerns, drug levels should be checked in mother and baby. Studies show that children who are breastfed have no adverse cognitive effects at 6 years of age.

- **Immunizations:** Most nursing mothers can be immunized routinely. Information is available on the Centers for Disease Control and Prevention Web site (see References on page 111). Examples of information available are

  - **Hepatitis A:** "Data on the safety of this vaccine in breastfeeding situations is not available. While it is unlikely that the vaccine would cause untoward effects in breastfed infants, consider administering immune globulin rather than vaccine."

  - **Rabies:** "Data concerning the safety of this vaccine for breastfeeding infants is not available. However, this vaccine is commonly given to nursing mothers without observed untoward effects in breastfed infants."

MATERNAL INGESTION OF FOODS AND HERBS (ADVICE ONLY) (MOTHER)

GENERAL CONSIDERATIONS

- **Prenatal Vitamins:** To ensure you are getting all recommended nutrients, it is a good idea to continue taking your prenatal vitamins while nursing.
- **Calcium:** You do not need to drink milk to make milk. As long as you are consuming the recommended daily amount of 1,000 mg in your diet (eg, cheese, yogurt, green leafy vegetables, calcium-fortified orange juice, milk), extra supplementation is not needed. You can lose 3% to 5% of your bone mass while breastfeeding, but within 6 months of weaning your body will resume normal bone mass.
- **Probiotics:** Taking *Lactobacillus fermentum* may be useful during breastfeeding as a strategy to prevent mastitis.
- **Foods You Usually Eat:** You should resume your normal diet and not specifically avoid categories of food or substances. There is no need to put unnecessary restrictions on your diet. Often foods believed to be bad in one culture, such as American (eg, garlic, chilies and other spicy foods, red peppers, lentils), are considered good for breastfeeding in another culture. If you ate the food during pregnancy, your baby may already be familiar with that taste, as the amniotic fluid is believed to share similar tastes with human milk.
- **Gassy Foods:** Watch your baby for unusual signs and symptoms (eg, unusual gassiness, explosive stools, persistent crying). If a food makes you gassy, such as cabbage, broccoli, beans, cauliflower, or onions, your baby may be affected. This gassiness should only be temporary.
- **Lactogenic Diets:** Lactogenic diets have been promoted as good for increasing milk supply. Recommendations include such foods as oatmeal, healthy fats (eg, olive oil), dark green vegetables, fennel, beets, and yams. Green papaya salads or soups are popular in Asia as a galactagogue. Eating the fruit while it is still green and full of papain enzyme is key. In some cultures (eg, Korean), seaweed soup is also thought to help with human milk production. Some cultures also recommend a protein soup with fish or chicken.
- **Nonalcoholic Malt and Ixbut Tea (*Euphorbia lancifolia*):** Have been used by Mayan Indians for centuries to help milk supply. Although no evidence supports that eating these foods increases milk, they all appear safe.
- **Fish and Mercury:** Fish provide omega-3 fatty acids and are a good source of protein. Caution should be taken with certain kinds of fish that may contain mercury because of the potential neurotoxic effects in babies. Albacore, ahi and bluefin tuna, pike, marlin, swordfish, shark, orange roughy, king mackerel, tilefish, and any fish caught in untested local waters should be avoided while nursing.
- **Herbs:** Herbs such as fenugreek, blessed thistle, alfalfa, red clover, and marshmallow root and drinking barley water have been touted as helpful for milk supply, yet there is limited high-quality evidence that these remedies increase milk supply.
- **Melatonin:** Melatonin is a natural hormone that is secreted in the brain and, if taken orally, can help with sleep. Little data exist on this, but it is unlikely that short-term use of usual doses of melatonin taken at night by a breastfeeding mother would adversely affect her infant.

Special Note: Take precautions in taking herbal preparations. Drink teas in moderation, check labels for all ingredients, and use a reliable brand, recognizing that these products are not regulated and, therefore, may not contain standard amounts of herbs. They may also contain other ingredients or contaminants that may not be safe. Lastly, concerns of allergies and interactions with other medications are increasing. Encourage mothers to look for GRAS herbs (ie, those that are generally regarded as safe by the US Food and Drug Administration).

See Other Protocol

- Lifestyle or Personal Care Questions (Advice Only) (for energy drinks) on page 54
- Maternal Medications (Advice Only) on page 67
- Substances of Abuse (Illicit Drugs) on page 99

MATERNAL MEDICATIONS (ADVICE ONLY) (MOTHER)

TRIAGE ASSESSMENT QUESTIONS

See Other Protocol
- Alcohol Use on page 1
- Substances of Abuse (Illicit Drugs) on page 99

GENERAL CONSIDERATIONS

In General, as a Breastfeeding Mother
- Avoid long-acting forms of medications.
- Try taking medication at time of or immediately following breastfeeding (best timing can depend on the medication).
- Watch your baby for unusual signs and symptoms (eg, sleepiness, irritability, other potential or known effects of the medication).
- When possible, encourage your doctor to choose a medication that will expose your baby to the least amount of it.

Pain Medications
- Acetaminophen (eg, Tylenol) and ibuprofen (eg, Advil, Motrin, Nuprin) are well studied and safe.
- Naproxen (eg, Naprosyn, Aleve) is longer acting and is safe for short-term use (eg, a few weeks).
- Aspirin (eg, Bayer) is secreted into human milk and has the potential to cause bleeding and Reye syndrome and should be avoided. However, baby aspirin (81 mg) taken daily for medical reasons by you (the mother) is allowable.
- In rare cases, mothers can be codeine hypermetabolizers, and this can be associated with sleepiness and apnea (stopping breathing) in breastfeeding babies.

Over-the-counter Medications
- Take care with over-the-counter medications that contain pseudoephedrine because it can decrease milk supply.
- Avoid combination products.
- Cough expectorants, such as Mucinex and Robitussin, have poor efficacy but no untoward effects in babies.

Low-Dose Aspirin
- Mothers with cardiovascular disease can reduce their risk by taking daily antiplatelet medications, such as low-dose aspirin (baby aspirin, 81 mg), which appears as a low-risk exposure to the infant in human milk.

Allergy Medications
- Diphenhydramine (eg, Benadryl) chlorpheniramine/brompheniramine (eg, Chlorphen, Chlor-Trimeton Allergy) can be sedating in babies so are not the best choice. Medications with less sedation include cetirizine (Zyrtec), loratadine (Claritin), and fexofenadine (Allegra).

Contraindicated Medications
- Concerns exist for amiodarone, chemotherapeutic/antineoplastic agents, chloramphenicol, ergotamine, gold salts, phenindione, radioactive pharmaceuticals, retinoids, tetracyclines (chronic >3 weeks), and certain psychotropic medications (lithium now can be taken with careful monitoring of blood levels in mother and baby).

ONLINE RESOURCES

Drugs and Lactation Database (LactMed)
- Located on the Toxnet Toxicology Data Network Web site of the US National Library of Medicine (www.toxnet.nlm.nih.gov/cgi-bin/sis/htmlgen?LACT), LactMed has information on use of medications during lactation, including an overall summary of use during breastfeeding, effects on breastfeeding and lactation, alternate medications to consider in breastfeeding women, drug levels in human milk, and references.

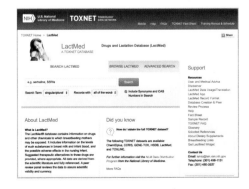

Texas Tech University Health Sciences Center
Infant Risk Center

- This site (www.infantrisk.com/categories/ breastfeeding) provides information about the safety of using prescribed and over-the-counter medications, herbal products, chemicals, vaccines, and other substances. It is particularly helpful for mothers on multiple medications. Warm line consultation telephone number: 800/352-2519 (Mon–Fri from 8:00 am–5:00 pm central time).

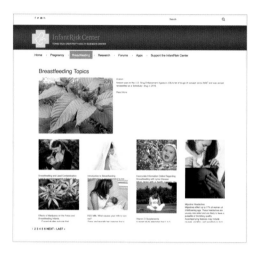

MATERNAL METHICILLIN-RESISTANT *STAPHYLOCOCCUS AUREUS* (MOTHER)

Definition

Mother has known cultured methicillin-resistant *Staphylococcus aureus* (MRSA) on an area of her body or on her breasts.

TRIAGE ASSESSMENT QUESTIONS

See Other Protocol

- Sore Nipples on page 93
- Breast Pain, Chronic >1 Week on page 9

See Today or Tomorrow in Office *(by Appointment)*

- Localized redness on skin surface or tenderness of breast
- Pain with palpation
  Reason: if mastitis, will need outpatient antibiotics

HOME CARE ADVICE

1 **Known MRSA in Non-breast Area:** Keep covered and continue to breastfeed. Practice good handwashing. MRSA does not pass into human milk.

2 **Known MRSA on Breast:** Feed on alternate side until lesions are healed; pump and discard milk on the affected side. Resume breastfeeding once treated with oral antibiotic (that covers MRSA) for 48 hours.

BACKGROUND INFORMATION

- MRSA is a bacterial infection that is resistant to numerous antibiotics, including methicillin, amoxicillin, penicillin, and oxacillin, causing difficulty in treatment of the infection.
- It can start as a minor skin sore, pimple, or boil but also become a more serious infection.
- Treatment options include clindamycin (may alter gastrointestinal flora or thrush), tetracyclines such as doxycycline and minocycline (short courses are safe when nursing but can also cause diarrhea and thrush), trimethoprim and sulfamethoxazole (should be avoided if newborn is younger than 4 weeks because of displacement of bilirubin or if infant has known glucose-6-phosphate dehydrogenase), and rifampin (best choice).

MATERNAL POSTPARTUM DEPRESSION (MOTHER)

Definition

- Feelings of sadness, anxiety, guilt, or worthlessness; difficulty sleeping despite being tired; weight change (loss or gain); or suicidal or infanticidal thoughts with onset within the first month postpartum.
- Also described as pregnancy-related depression or mood disorder.
- Screening using a standardized tool such as the 10-question Edinburgh Postnatal Depression Scale (EPDS) is recommended in the pediatrician's office or by the mother's physician.

TRIAGE ASSESSMENT QUESTIONS

Go to ED Now (or to Office With PCP Approval)

⬤ Mother has thoughts of harming herself or baby
Reason: if mother reports intent or plan to hurt herself or others, wanting to die, or hallucinations, she will need to be hospitalized for treatment; call the mother's obstetrician or primary care physician to alert him or her to the mother's severe symptoms

See Other Protocol

⬤ Maternal Medications (Advice Only) on page 67
⬤ Emotional Symptoms With Letdown on page 24
⬤ Breastfeeding in the First Few Weeks: Simplify Your Life (Advice Only) on page 10

See Today or Tomorrow in Office (by Appointment)

⬤ May come up as part of initial screening, or triage practitioner may need to have a high index of suspicion
⬤ Symptoms from day 2 through day 10 classified as baby blues; day 11 and beyond classified as postpartum depression
⬤ If positive response to any of the following conditions, can refer mother to her obstetrician or primary care physician for depression screening
Reason: if concern for any of these questions is present, mother may need formal postnatal counseling and treatment EPDS (10 questions)

- Sad or miserable
- Crying a lot
- Difficulty sleeping even though tired
- Poor appetite
- Feelings of worthlessness, guilt, or blame
- Feeling anxious, worried, scared, or panicky
- Overwhelmed

Home Care

○ Baby blues, started at day 2 to 3 (Range is days 2–10.)
○ Mother feeling tired and emotional

HOME CARE ADVICE

❶ **Reassurance:** Baby blues usually start at 2 to 3 days after birth and last until about 10 days.

❷ **Sleep and Maternal Self-care:** Lack of sleep can make new mothers more emotional. Try to get some protected sleep, and ask for help from your partner or spouse, family, or friends.

❸ **Call Back If:** Advice not helping. If you follow home care advice, see within 3 days in office (by appointment).

BACKGROUND INFORMATION

- Depressed mothers have been shown to have more difficulty with breastfeeding, and studies indicate that exclusive breastfeeding in the early months is negatively associated with postpartum depressive symptoms.
- Need to support breastfeeding because it may be the only thing that the depressed mother feels is going well, and weaning early may lead to more feelings of guilt.
- Need to identify postpartum depression for mother's and baby's health because babies of untreated mothers with depression are more likely to have neurobehavioral delays at 1 year of age.

Causes

- Postpartum depression is the most common psychiatric illness in new mothers, with prevalence of 10% to 20%.

- More mothers experience the baby blues, with prevalence as high as 40% to 80%.
- Some women have had similar symptoms in pregnancy.
- Baby blues is associated with fall in hormones at 3 to 7 days' postpartum.
- Postpartum psychosis is rare and occurs in 1 out of 1,000 births. These mothers are delusional and agitated and have unusual thoughts or hallucinations.

Treatment Options

- Cognitive-behavioral or interpersonal psychotherapy may be enough for some mothers.
- However, other mothers may need a prescription medication trial.
- First-line selective serotonin reuptake inhibitors such as sertraline (Zoloft), paroxetine (Paxil), and escitalopram (Lexapro), are best because their levels are very low in human milk.
- Fluoxetine (Prozac) is not preferred because of its longer half-life and associated higher levels in human milk.
- However, if mother has had a good response to fluoxetine and other medications have not been helpful, baby can breastfeed and be followed for any potential adverse effects.

MATERNAL POSTPARTUM VAGINAL BLEEDING (MOTHER)

Definition

- Postpartum bleeding may increase with breastfeeding and oxytocin release because the uterus contracts more rapidly. It ultimately decreases the mother's overall bleeding and leads to lower levels of postpartum hemorrhage and anemia.
- More serious bleeding (eg, postpartum hemorrhage due to retained placenta), if not addressed appropriately, can have long-term consequences for mother's milk supply.

TRIAGE ASSESSMENT QUESTIONS

Go to ED Now *(or to Office With PCP Approval)*

● Increase in frequency of vaginal bleeding or larger clots, changing feminine pads more than every 2 hours
  Reason: concern for serious causes of postpartum bleeding
● Increasing or continuous abdominal pain
  Reason: uterine trauma or infection
● Temperature above 100.5°F (38.1°C)
  Reason: uterine infection
● Dizziness or feeling light-headed
  Reason: symptomatic from loss of blood
● Malodorous vaginal discharge
  Reason: uterine infection

See Other Protocol

◉ Maternal Illnesses (Advice Only) on page 64

Home Care

○ Reference range amounts of postpartum bleeding using one feminine pad every 3 hours
○ Clots passed that are smaller than a small plum or apricot sized

HOME CARE ADVICE

❶ **Rest Assured (for Normal Bleeding Pattern):** Nursing mothers often feel uterine contractions with nursing and may sense simultaneous bleeding as a result. Normal bleeding consists of a few days of bright red bleeding, and then rust or colored bleeding in first few days postpartum, only using one feminine pad every 3 hours. Clots smaller than a small plum or apricot sized are normal even though these can be alarming.

❷ **Practice Maternal Self-care:** No heavy lifting is recommended in the first 6 weeks. You may notice increased bleeding if increasing physical activity.

❸ **Call Your Own Doctor for Continued Concerns:** If continued concerns, call your own primary care physician, or the obstetrician-gynecologist who delivered your baby, to arrange evaluation.

BACKGROUND INFORMATION

Causes of Postpartum Bleeding

- Increased uterine contractions with nursing.
- Genital tract trauma from cesarean delivery, forceps or vacuum delivery, or newborn with macrosomia.
- Uterine infection or chorioamnionitis.
- Uterine atony (uterine muscle not contracting).
- Retained placental fragments should be suspected as a cause, especially if mother has unexplained low milk supply.
- May need help advocating for a uterine ultrasound.
- Thrombocytopenia, coagulation disorders, or other inherited bleeding dysfunction (eg, von Willebrand disease).

MATERNAL SMOKING, VAPING, AND CESSATION STRATEGIES (MOTHER)

Definition

- Tobacco exposure through inhalation of cigarettes concomitant with breastfeeding.
- Vaping or use of e-cigarettes has not been studied in breastfeeding mothers so use of these as a strategy to decrease nicotine use should be cautioned.

TRIAGE ASSESSMENT QUESTIONS

Go to ED Now *(or to Office With PCP Approval)*

● Smoking and using cessation nicotine (ie, doing both)
Reason: worrisome because of nicotine effect on baby

● Baby jittery or restless
Reason: could be a nicotine adverse effect

● Baby with vomiting or diarrhea
Reason: could be a nicotine adverse effect

See Within 3 Days in Office *(by Appointment)*

◗ Mother ready to discuss smoking cessation

Home Care

○ Smoking from one cigarette to up to a pack per day (Less is better, of course.)
○ Using any smoking cessation medications (eg, gum, patch)

HOME CARE ADVICE

❶ **Try to Breastfeed and Quit Smoking:** Consider smoking cessation assistance. Secondhand smoke exposure is associated with other toxins, such as carbon monoxide and cyanide. Any non-inhaled nicotine is better for your baby than smoking.

❷ **If You Cannot Quit, Cut Down:** If it is not possible to quit, decrease the number of cigarettes or try ones that are low in nicotine. Delay feeding as long as possible after smoking. Smoke cigarettes outside, and do not smoke around your baby.

❸ **Consider Cessation Medications:** Most states have a quit line, and many insurances cover smoking cessation treatments. Safe options for breastfeeding mothers include
- **Smoking a Few Cigarettes per Day:** Use Nicorette gum.
- **Smoking 1 Pack per Day:** Use nicotine patch.
- **Smoking More Than 1 Pack per Day:** Use bupropion. Bupropion doses of up to 300 mg daily produce low levels of nicotine in human milk and should not cause adverse effects in breastfed infants, but there is little reported use in breastfed newborns. Cases have been reported of a possible seizure in partially breastfed 6-month-olds.
- **Vaping:** Vaping and e-cigarettes contain nicotine and the vapor may contain toxic substances such as hydrocarbons. Since e-cigarettes are not licensed or regulated, it is best for the nursing mother to use other options for nicotine replacement therapy and smoking cessation. The aerosol released contains nicotine and other toxic chemicals, so infants should be kept away from the vapor.
Note: Adverse effects of the patch include nightmares.
Note: Adverse effects of bupropion include depressive symptoms and seizures.

BACKGROUND INFORMATION

- Many women stop smoking in pregnancy but relapse after the birth of their baby.
- Mothers who smoke are less likely to breastfeed.
- Effects of smoking on the risk of sudden infant death syndrome and respiratory illness are almost negated if the baby has been breastfed.
- Nicotine interferes with letdown and can be associated with lower milk supply.
- Smoking between 10 and 20 cigarettes a day results in nicotine levels of 0.4 and 0.5 mg/L in human milk; this correlates with adverse effects (eg, jitteriness) seen in the baby.

MILK LEAKING FROM NEWBORN'S BREASTS (GALACTORRHEA) (BABY, EARLY)

Definition

- Milk or colostrum leaking from newborn's breasts
- Often associated with breast buds
- Called "witch's milk" in the 1850s during a time of witchcraft when fear led to misunderstood things being attributed to witches

TRIAGE ASSESSMENT QUESTIONS

Home Care

○ Newborn who has breast buds that are leaking milk
○ Newborn who also has swollen labia or vaginal discharge or blood

HOME CARE ADVICE

Reassurance: Leaking milk or vaginal bloody discharge in the newborn is a biological response to maternal hormones and should resolve in a few weeks to months.

BACKGROUND INFORMATION

- Absorption of hormones from mother causes stimulation of breast tissue in newborn.

MILK STORAGE AND RETURN TO WORK/SCHOOL (MILK EXPRESSION)

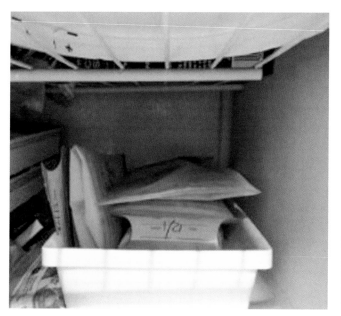

Milk storage in regular freezer

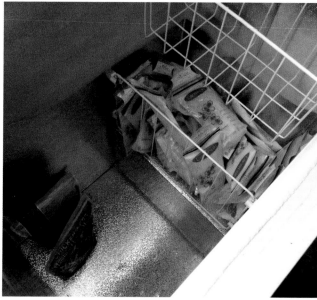

Milk storage in a deep freezer

Definition

- Expression of human milk during times of mother-baby separation for provision of milk for feeding at a later time
- Separation of mother and baby for periods longer than 4 hours
- Temporary maternal issues that required milk expression and storage

TRIAGE ASSESSMENT QUESTIONS

See Other Protocol

- Exclusive Pumping on page 27
- Expression of Human Milk: Pumping, Parts and Cleaning Equipment, Hand Expression (Advice Only) on page 29

Home Care

- ○ Returning to work or school
- ○ Has not talked with employer yet
- ○ Needs advice about pumping and storage

HOME CARE ADVICE

❶ Meet With Your Supervisor: Set up a meeting to talk with your supervisor about your desire to pump at work and the need for a private place. Ideally, this should occur before your maternity leave begins. If possible, it may be better to work part-time and start midpoint of the first week back. Federal legislation requires employers to have a private place (not a bathroom stall) and to accommodate reasonable break times for pumping milk.

❷ Make a Plan—the Sooner the Better: Think about how you will plan your workday and site, such as cubicle, office, or other place to pump. Watch "Breastfeeding and Working" YouTube videos (www.cobfc.org) and read *Milk Memos* (see References on page 111) to assist with this planning.

❸ Get a Good Pump and Storage Bags: Double-sided electric breast pump is best for working mothers. Resealable milk storage bags can be purchased at most baby supply stores. Some mothers prefer to store in glass bottles. Containers made with bisphenol A should be avoided.

❹ **Set It All Up Before Starting Workday:** Setting up the whole system at the start of your shift or in advance of your break is helpful because it saves time that can be used for pumping.

❺ **Good Handwashing and Cleaning of Parts:** Always wash your hands before pumping. Parts that come in contact with the breast or human milk should be cleaned as soon as possible after pumping. Use running water and do not place pump parts in the sink.

❻ **Have a Personal Cooler for Human Milk Storage:** It is easier to store milk in a cooler than to try to store it in a community-used refrigerator with others' lunches. Human milk will keep for 8 hours in a cooler with an ice pack. This milk should be consumed in the next few days.

❼ **Use Rule of 4s:** Guidelines for milk storage are easy to remember: 4 hours at room temperature, 4 days in the refrigerator, and, actually, 6 months or even longer in the freezer. Previously thawed frozen milk should be used within 24 hours and not left out at room temperature for more than 2 hours. These are the conservative limits (Table). Always use oldest frozen milk first, and thaw in refrigerator or hot water. Never use the microwave; the temperature differential not only is dangerous for babies but also can destroy some proteins.

❽ **Eat Fresh:** Fresh or refrigerated human milk is better than frozen (to help keep immune properties intact). If freezing milk, it should be done as soon as possible after pumping.

❾ **Pumping in the Morning Is Best for Your Stockpile:** Pump first thing in early morning (after first feeding; wait 1 hour) to have an extra supply at home because milk supply is greatest at that time.

❿ **Practice 15 for 4:** You need to express milk for 15 minutes, on average, for each 4 hours that you are away from your baby.

⓫ **Meet Up With Baby:** May help you avoid a pumping session and allow you to reconnect with your baby.

⓬ **Reverse-Cycle Nursing Can Occur:** Sometimes babies do not eat when the mother is away and wait to nurse when she returns (they eat frequently during the night and take longer sleep stretches during the day). This phenomenon can be difficult for many mothers, though some mothers enjoy it because they feel connected to their babies. Ask caregivers to try to offer a sippy cup or solids if this appears to be the pattern and your babies is at the appropriate maturity level (ie, at least 4–6 months of age).

BACKGROUND INFORMATION

- Most mothers return to work or school within 2 months postpartum.
- Part-time working mothers who are at home breastfeed longer than full-time working mothers (ie, duration of breastfeeding is affected by employment).
- Human milk storage is a safe and healthy option for mothers who require separation from their babies because of return to work or school or other factors.

Table. Suggested Guidelines for Milk Storage and Use for All Infants

Storage Method and Temperature	Maximum Amount of Time for Storage
Room (16°C–29°C [60.8°F–84.2°F])	4 h optimal (6–8 h acceptable under very clean conditions)
Refrigerator (4°C [39.2°F])	96 h 4 d optimal (5–8 d under very clean conditions)
Previously thawed refrigerated milk	24 h
Freezer (−17.8°C [0°F])	6 mo optimal (12 mo acceptable)

Modified from American Academy of Pediatrics, American College of Obstetricians and Gynecologists. *Breastfeeding Handbook for Physicians.* Schanler RJ, Krebs NF, Mass SB, eds. 2nd ed. Elk Grove Village, IL: American Academy of Pediatrics; 2014:170.

MISTAKEN MILK INGESTION, MILK SHARING (SPECIAL CIRCUMSTANCES)

Definition

- Child is mistakenly fed another child's bottle of expressed human milk (bottle switch in child care setting); should be treated as an unintentional exposure to bodily fluids.
- Informal and formal milk sharing is a growing practice, and early evidence is concerning because little is known about maternal factors as well as associated bacterial contamination.

TRIAGE ASSESSMENT QUESTIONS

See Today in Office *(by Appointment)*

- Child should undergo baseline test for HIV
- Mother whose milk was ingested should be encouraged to share any prenatal test results with mother of exposed child
  Reason: this can be reassuring to mother of exposed child while awaiting test results

BACKGROUND INFORMATION

- Donor milk from a certified milk bank has become more available and is used in some birth hospitals for early preterm and term newborns. Barriers include cost and lack of access. Mothers may view its use as a short-term approach to supplementation and will perhaps be more likely to return to exclusively breastfeeding.
- Risk of HIV transmission from human milk is low because women in the United States who are HIV positive are advised to not breastfeed.
- Transmission from a single human milk exposure has never been documented.
- Informal milk sharing is common with relatives and friends.
- Formal milk sharing on the Internet is concerning, with one study showing that 75% of cases involved milk contaminated with bacteria.

MULTIPLES (ADVICE ONLY) (SPECIAL CIRCUMSTANCES)

GENERAL CONSIDERATIONS

- Attempt to get babies to breastfeed at the same time (tandem) as soon as possible.
- At first, you may want to breastfeed one at a time to give each baby time to learn and allow yourself to get comfortable with breastfeeding.
- Breastfeeding multiples can be associated with more difficulties, including maternal fatigue, mental health issues, delayed milk coming in, insufficient milk, and latch and positioning problems.
- However, many mothers can breastfeed multiples with minimal to no breastfeeding difficulty and will make more milk to meet their babies' needs. Some mothers of multiples make up to 3 L of milk per day!
- Sixty percent of twins and 90% of higher-order multiples are born at fewer than 37 weeks' gestation. These babies are at risk of having feeding difficulty because of preterm birth and other medical complications.
- Time is the biggest deterrent for mothers of multiples.
- You should ask for and get as much help as soon as possible.
- When you are beyond the first month postpartum, you may want to connect with your local chapter of Multiples of America (formerly known as the National Organization of Mothers of Twins Clubs) (www.multiplesofamerica.org).

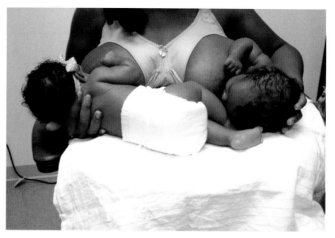

Tandem breastfeeding of twins: cross cradle and football/clutch hold combination positions

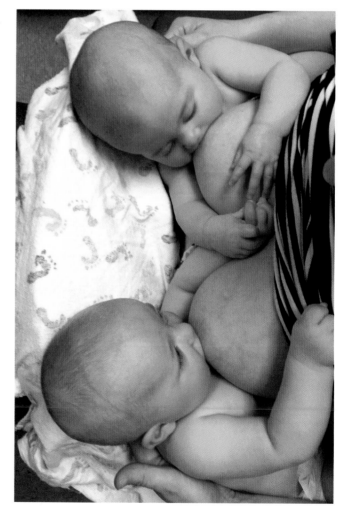

Tandem nursing of 6-month-old twins in the football/clutch position

NEWBORN CONTRAINDICATIONS TO BREASTFEEDING (ADVICE ONLY) (SPECIAL CIRCUMSTANCES)

GENERAL CONSIDERATIONS

- Many inherited disorders present as failure to thrive, and newborns, therefore, are often weaned in the process of diagnosis, which is not always appropriate.

Absolute Contraindication

Galactosemia
- Known galactosemia is confirmed on newborn screening results in most states by detecting a decreased galactose 1-phosphate uridyltransferase level. Galactosemia is one of the true newborn contraindications to breastfeeding.
- Newborn is unable to metabolize sugar, such as the lactose/galactose in human milk (also bovine milk formula).
- Newborn may continue breastfeeding while awaiting confirmatory testing (blood and urine tests), but this should occur in discussion with her primary care physician.
- If the baby is supplementing, this should occur with lactose-free soy formulas.
- With galactosemia, babies can appear well initially but will develop signs of lethargy, poor feeding, jaundice, liver disease, coagulopathy, and sepsis when galactose levels build too high.

BREASTFEED WITH CAUTION AND ONLY UNDER DIRECTION OF A MEDICAL PROVIDER EXPERT IN THE CONDITION.

Phenylketonuria
A metabolic disorder known as phenylketonuria, or PKU, is also diagnosed on newborn screening results and is a partial contraindication to breastfeeding. These babies will need to feed on a special low-phenylalanine diet.
- Because human milk is lower in phenylalanine than bovine milk formula, mothers can usually continue breastfeeding while supplementing their baby's diet with a low-phenylalanine formula. Weight gain and phenylalanine levels should be followed closely in these babies.

- Careful monitoring of phenylalanine levels in the blood is essential with intake of human milk.

Cystic Fibrosis
- Newborns with cystic fibrosis should breastfeed along with pancreatic enzymes and will benefit from infection protection.

Extreme Preterm Birth
- Newborns born extremely preterm may not be able to breastfeed initially at the breast but can benefit from receiving pumped milk. These babies may require vitamins or other supplements.

NIPPLE ABNORMALITY: FLAT/SHORT, INVERTED, LARGE, OR BULBOUS (MOTHER)

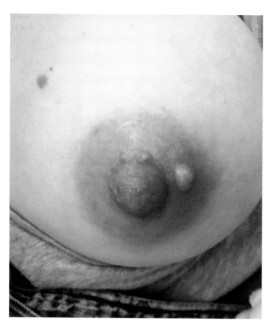

Enlarged non-tender Montgomery gland surrounding the nipple

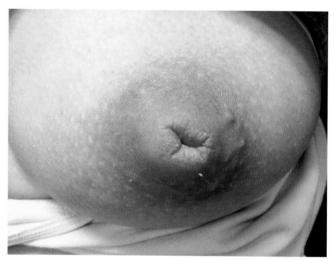

Inverted nipple

Definition

Abnormality of the nipple that may pose difficulty with breastfeeding, such as flat, inverted, unusual, or bulbous in shape or large in proportion to baby's mouth

TRIAGE ASSESSMENT QUESTIONS

See Other Protocol

- No Latch or Inability to Latch on page 82
- Low Milk Supply on page 57
- Engorgement on page 25

See Within 3 Days in Office *(by Appointment)*

- Concern that milk supply is compromised by ineffective latch

Home Care

- ○ Nipples with a different configuration—flat/short, inverted, large/long, Tootsie Roll, or gumball shaped
- ○ Breasts edematous after delivery and causing flatness of nipple

HOME CARE ADVICE

❶ **Flat/Short Nipples:** Latch is compromised because your baby needs the nipple to be placed further back in his mouth in the early weeks to maintain latch. He can also slide off the breast more easily. Try using manual or electric breast pump stimulation of nipples, attempting to get them more erect prior to latching on.

❷ **Inverted Nipples:** Inverted nipples cause the same phenomenon as flat nipples but may be more difficult to bring to a more erect position with stimulation. Try a syringe or an electric breast pump to bring your nipples out. Wearing breast shells does not appear to be effective in helping mothers evert their nipples. They are considered cumbersome and are no longer recommended.

❸ **Large/Long, Tootsie Roll–Shaped, or Gumball-Shaped Nipples:** This kind of mouth and nipple mismatch is problematic because your baby gets a mouthful of nipple and cannot adequately stimulate milk ducts. With this issue, mothers usually need more assistance with latch. Pumping until your baby's mouth gets big enough to handle the nipple is usually necessary. Be assured that your nipple will not grow, but your baby's mouth will!

❹ **Pump:** May need to pump to maintain milk supply until latch evaluation is possible.

❺ **Edema of Breasts:** If edema of breasts, may need to do reverse flow maneuver.
Note: See Engorgement protocol on page 25 for instructions.

❻ **Nipple Shield:** Although nipple shields can be bought over the counter, they should be used with a lactation specialist or physician supervision. Often fitting or stuffing the nipple into the nipple shield makes it manageable for your baby to latch, stay on, and transfer milk more effectively.

❼ **Call Back If:** Advice not helping. See within 3 days in office (by appointment).

BACKGROUND INFORMATION

- Nipples come in different configurations. Many can breastfeed without difficulties. However, some mothers will not have been made aware that this may cause them breastfeeding difficulty.
- As babies get older and their mouths get bigger, most will overcome the nipple shape abnormality.
- Flat/short nipples cause the baby to have trouble latching, and the baby slides or comes off with feedings.
- Edematous areola results from intravenous oxytocin or large amounts of intravenous fluid given to mothers in labor.
- Inverted nipples are nipples that are turned outside in (see photo on previous page).
- Large/long nipples are ones that are out of proportion with a baby's mouth size. The mother's nipples can be long like a Tootsie Roll or round like a gumball, and this can make nursing difficult in the first month until the baby's mouth gets bigger with age.

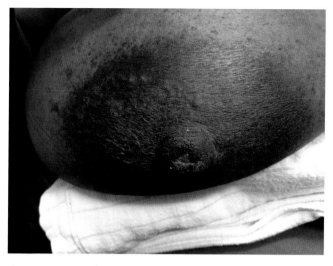

Generous nipple size can cause difficulty with latch or milk transfer. (Nipple shown is >2 cm.)

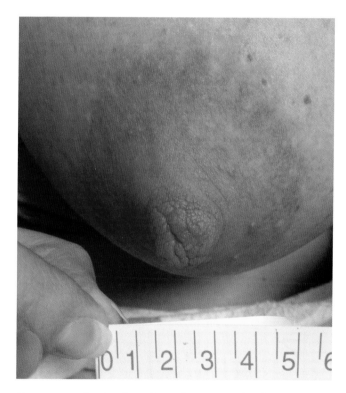

Generous nipple size >2 cm (average nipple size is 1.3 cm).

NO LATCH OR INABILITY TO LATCH (BABY, EARLY)

Definition

Baby is not latching on and cries or acts distressed when put to breast, or he does not seem to know what to do when breast is offered.

TRIAGE ASSESSMENT QUESTIONS

See Other Protocol

- Exclusive Pumping on page 27
- Breast Pain (engorgement) on page 6
- Nipple Abnormality: Flat/Short, Inverted, Large, or Bulbous on page 80
- Pacifiers and Slow-Flow Nipples (Advice Only) on page 88

See Today in Office *(by Appointment)*

If these items were not instituted in the hospital before discharge, a more urgent evaluation is indicated.

- Baby never latched in the birth hospital
- Nipples are flat/short, inverted, or large/long for baby's mouth (Unfortunately, mother may not be aware of any abnormality.)
  Reason: see physician or lactation specialist for feeding evaluation, assistance with obtaining a breast pump, or trial with a Supplemental Nursing System (see photo on next page) or nipple shield

Home Care

- ○ Nipple/flow confusion (Baby received formula in a bottle in the birth hospital.)
- ○ Unsure if bottle has slow-flow nipple; may be easier for baby with fast flow
- ○ Engorged breasts and infant cannot latch on

HOME CARE ADVICE

❶ **Review Latch:** Relax and talk to your baby. Try tickling her upper lip with nipple, waiting for her mouth to open wide, and latching her on with nipple aiming to roof of mouth.

❷ **Consider Nipple Confusion:** Twenty-five percent of babies develop a bottle preference when it is introduced before 3 to 4 weeks of age. Eventually, your baby will get back on track, but you may need assistance from a lactation consultant, use of a Supplemental Nursing System at the breast with supplemental milk for extra flow, or temporary use of a nipple shield.

❸ **Check for Slow Flow:** If your baby is using a bottle, use a slow-flow nipple. At times, even nipples labeled as slow flow drip readily once the bottle is tipped upside down.

❹ **Perform Finger Trick or Bait and Switch:** Try having your baby suck on your (or another caregiver's) finger first to calm your baby and organize suck, and trick her by switching over to the breast.

❺ **Place Skin to Skin:** This can help get an uninterested baby back on track. It also helps with your milk letdown and may help with your milk supply. Put your baby skin to skin about 15 to 30 minutes prior to anticipated feeding to assist with latch.

❻ **Hand Express Milk:** Perform breast massage and hand expression prior to feeding to allow your baby to smell or taste your milk.

❼ **Perform Reverse-Pressure Softening Technique:** Gentle 2-handed pressure on the breast to push edema away from the areola may help your baby latch better.

❽ **Pump:** Continue to express milk every 2 to 3 hours if no latch is possible. Use the milk to drip onto your nipples at start of the feeding to cue your baby to where milk is found.

❾ **Call Back If:** Advice not helping. See within 3 days in office (by appointment).

BACKGROUND INFORMATION

- Concerns about refusal to breastfeed should always trigger concerns about a sick baby.
- Breast-mouth mismatch (ie, large breast, small mouth) is difficult to discern by phone.
- Baby will readily take a bottle and has developed confusion between bottle and breastfeeding. Early preference can occur and has been called *nipple confusion* because it appears easier for baby to get milk from bottle because of flow differences. *Important: Preference for bottle is not because baby likes formula better or does not want to breastfeed.*

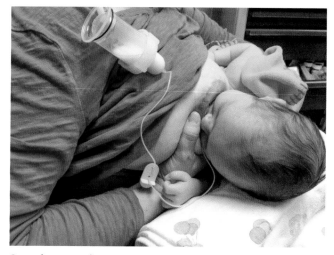

Supplemental Nursing System in use

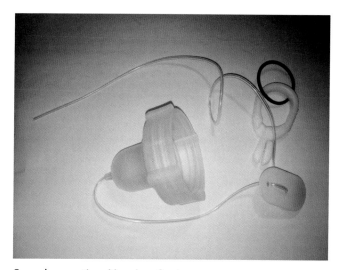

Supplementing Nursing System

NURSING STRIKE OR REFUSAL (BABY, EARLY)

Definition

Temporary refusal of nursing when breast is offered to baby; most often occurs at 3 to 4 months

TRIAGE ASSESSMENT QUESTIONS

See Other Protocol

- Exclusive Pumping on page 27
- Milk Storage and Return to Work/School on page 75

Home Care

- ○ Return of mother's menstrual period recently
- ○ New maternal soaps, perfumes, or deodorants
- ○ Maternal stressors
- ○ Signs or symptoms of illness in baby—congestion, fever, seems to have pain in the mouth
- ○ Teething behaviors—fussiness, increased hands in mouth and rubbing gums, increased drooling
- ○ Any unusual foods eaten by mother 8 to 12 hours before nursing (eg, garlic, onion, even mint candies)
- ○ Developmental events with infant aged 4 to 5 months, 7 months, or 9 to 12 months; infant more recently interested in environment and complementary foods
- ○ Preference for only one breast at a time

HOME CARE ADVICE

❶ **Reassurance:** Nursing strike or refusal usually resolves; deciphering the cause can be challenging.

❷ **Changes With Mother**
- Return of menstrual period may cause a temporary drop in milk.
- Any other changes going on with you can be sensed by your baby and may result in nursing refusal (eg, new soap, perfume, deodorant, stress, unusual foods).

❸ **Changes in Baby:** May be related to teething or is early sign of illness or certain developmental milestones.

❹ **Concern for Baby Hydration:** May offer sippy cup or bottle.

❺ **Pump:** Express milk during period of refusal and store for later.

❻ **Hand Express or Pump for Quicker Letdown:** May help to get milk reward to baby faster.

❼ **Trying at Sleepy Time or in the Bathtub:** May be helpful to offer some expressed human milk before trying to nurse because the baby may be more patient to work on breastfeeding if less hungry. Offer the breast when your baby is sleepier or in a totally different location (eg, the bathtub can be a relaxing and unusual place to nurse).

❽ **Nursing One Side Only Is Norm:** Most babies worldwide settle into nursing just one side or breast at a time.

❾ **Call Back If:** Advice not helping; if behavior does not change, see within 3 days in office (by appointment).

BACKGROUND INFORMATION

- Return of mother's menstrual period can cause a temporary drop in milk supply.
- May be first sign that baby is ill (eg, earache, nasal congestion, throat lesions).
- Refusal can also occur with other teething behaviors.
- Strong-tasting foods eaten by mother 8 to 12 hours earlier (eg, garlic, onion, even mint candies).
- Change in maternal soap, perfume, or deodorant or new stressors in mother.
- Preference for one breast is common, but total refusal of one breast may be a sign of disease in that breast.
- May follow an episode of biting mother, and baby was startled by mother's reaction.
- Occasionally, a nipple shield may help with transitioning to the breast, so a visit with a lactation specialist may be warranted.
- If older infant, may be window for child-led weaning.

NURSING WITH PREGNANCY (SPECIAL CIRCUMSTANCES)

Definition
Mother is nursing her baby, toddler, or child and becomes pregnant.

TRIAGE ASSESSMENT QUESTIONS

See Other Protocol
- Sore Nipples on page 93

See Today or Tomorrow in Office *(by Appointment)*
- Preterm labor risk or contractions this pregnancy
- History of previous miscarriages
- Bleeding
- Weight loss or struggling to gain weight this pregnancy
- Vegan or have any other dietary restrictions
  Reason: need to discuss with own doctor risk of continuing nursing

Home Care
- ○ Nausea with nursing
- ○ Agitated with nursing
- ○ Decrease in milk supply

HOME CARE ADVICE

❶ **Relaxation Techniques:** Try deep breathing or distraction when nursing to help with pain or nausea symptoms.

❷ **Decrease in Supply:** May go unnoticed by your baby/child but may also lead to frustration at the breast. This depends on age. Some older children adjust to change. Because this decrease in supply is hormonally mediated, usual methods to increase milk supply may not be working.

❸ **Call Back If:** Advice not helping. See within 3 days in office (by appointment).

BACKGROUND INFORMATION
- Some mothers experience discomfort with nursing (ie, sore nipples and a decrease in milk supply midpregnancy [20 weeks]).
- Others experience some agitation or nausea with letdown.
- Hormonal changes, such as higher estrogen levels with pregnancy, can affect hormone levels for nursing, so about two-thirds experience a decrease in milk supply.
- Because of these symptoms, about 25% of mothers end up weaning their infant/child when they get pregnant.

OVERACTIVE LETDOWN/OVERABUNDANT MILK SUPPLY (BABY, EARLY)

Definition
Overactive letdown in early postpartum period can cause baby to pull away from breast and cry or choke and sputter. This also can occur at other times with mothers who have overabundant milk supply.

TRIAGE ASSESSMENT QUESTIONS

See Other Protocol
- Gassiness in the Breastfed Baby on page 44
- Fussiness, Colic, and Crying in the Breastfed Baby on page 41
- Breast Pain (plugged duct prevention) on page 6
- Tandem Nursing on page 100

Home Care
- ○ Leaking milk, frequently engorged, or full even after a good feeding
- ○ Painful sensations with letdown
- ○ Baby who cries, coughs, pulls away, or all of the above after a few minutes of nursing
- ○ Baby who has increased gas or explosive greenish stools

HOME CARE ADVICE

❶ Rest Assured: Some mothers with overabundant milk supply may have painful sensations with letdown, and deep-breathing relaxation techniques can help. You may also need to wear cloth breast pads with a bra for leaking milk.

❷ Try Laid-back Nursing: Try to feed your baby leaning back on a sofa or comfy chair to get assistance from gravity so that the squirt of milk with letdowns will be less forceful. Your baby will have more control over flow in this position.

❸ Take a Break: You should interrupt feeding and let your baby recover, waiting until the spray of milk stops. You may need to pause numerous times within a nursing session.

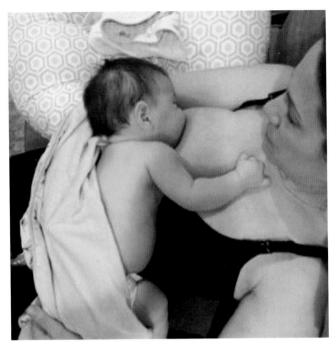

Leaning-back position offers advantage that baby is 'on top of the breast.'

❹ Pump Off the Foremilk: To help decrease foremilk as well as volume your baby may get at the start of feedings, pump off the foremilk (first 5 minutes). Label and save this milk for later; you may need to eventually mix it with other pumped milk.

❺ Offer Only One Breast per Feed: Best to move to one-sided feedings: allow your baby to finish one side completely; only pump off the undrained side if needed for comfort purposes. This practice allows your baby to get more hindmilk (higher fat, slower gastric emptying) and allows better digestion of lactose from foremilk. With time, you should see a decrease in green, foamy stools.

❻ Avoid Pumping to Stockpile: Avoid increased pumping at this time, as this will only encourage increased milk supply. Use pump only for comfort when needed. You can start pumping to stockpile later when you have worked through issues of overabundant supply.

❼ **Call Back If:** Advice not helping. See within 3 days in office (by appointment).

BACKGROUND INFORMATION

- Spray of milk at initiation of a feeding occurs primarily in primipara mothers.
- It can occur in multiparous mothers who have overabundance of milk supply, are tandem nursing, or are "über-pumpers."

PACIFIERS AND SLOW-FLOW NIPPLES (ADVICE ONLY) (BABY, EARLY)

GENERAL CONSIDERATIONS

Pacifiers

- Avoid pacifiers in the first few weeks until breast-feeding is well established.
- Pacifiers can lead to missed feeding cues. If deemed necessary, pacifier may be offered as long as it has not been 90 minutes since last nursing session.
- Pacifiers may lead to shorter overall duration of breastfeeding.
- However, there are circumstances (eg, high suck need in babies with prenatal drug exposure or preterm birth, painful procedures, multiples) in which they can be helpful if correct guidance is provided for their use.
- Round nipple–type pacifier is preferable to others because the shape is closer to a mother's nipple shape.
- After the first few weeks, mothers can use pacifiers for urgent situations, such as a baby screaming uncontrollably in the car or on an airplane, or evening crying or colic if baby is not hungry. Pacifiers have been associated with sudden infant death syndrome reduction for sleep at night, but how this works is unclear.
- Pacifiers may protect against early cessation of exclusive breastfeeding among mothers at risk for postpartum depression. More research is needed to explore this association.

Slow-Flow Nipples and Bottles

- Slow-flow nipples should always be used when supplementing. Bottle nipple can be evaluated for slow flow by turning bottle upside down to make sure that no drops of milk come out without squeezing the nipple itself.
- Fast-flow bottle-feedings may result in baby preference for bottle and frustration at the breast.
  Note: Caution should be taken with advising about bottle nipples. Some nipples may be labeled as slow flow but are not. Author's experience is that Philips Avent and Medela brands are the most reliable.

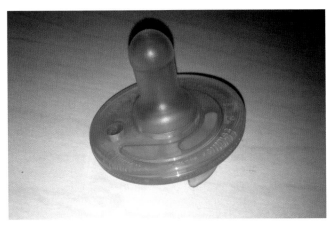

Newer version of round nipple–type pacifier

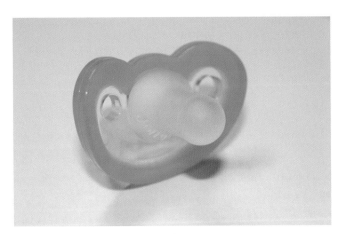

Rounded nipple–type pacifier

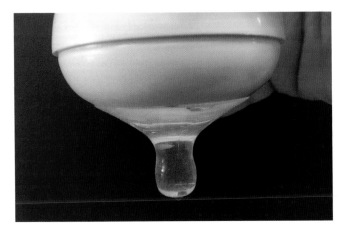

Testing a slow-flow bottle by inverting it and watching for minimal drops

REFERRAL TO LOCAL RESOURCES (ADVICE ONLY) (MOTHER)

(Insert your own local numbers here for breastfeeding community contacts.)

_____

_____

American Academy of Pediatrics Chapter Breastfeeding Coordinators

www.aap.org/en-us/advocacy-and-policy/aap-health-initiatives/Breastfeeding/Pages/Chapter-Breastfeeding-Coordinators-Roster.aspx

The American Academy of Pediatrics is a national organization of pediatricians with designated physician liaisons who are experts in lactation as well as connected in their communities. These chapter breastfeeding coordinators can be helpful for recommending referral resources.

_____

_____

Special Supplemental Nutrition Program for Women, Infants, and Children State Breastfeeding Information and Locations

www.fns.usda.gov/wic

The Special Supplemental Nutrition Program for Women, Infants, and Children provides federal grants to states for supplemental foods, health care referrals, and nutrition education for low-income pregnant, breastfeeding, and non-breastfeeding postpartum women, as well as to infants and children up to age 5 years who are found to be at nutritional risk.

_____

_____

International Lactation Consultant Association

www.ilca.org

The International Lactation Consultant Association is for lactation consultants, health care professionals who have special training in helping mothers with lactation. It has a bookstore, position papers, and information about conferences. It also allows one to search for lactation consultants by zip code.

_____

_____

Hospital Breastfeeding Follow-up Sites

_____

_____

Other Outpatient Follow-up Sites

_____

_____

Breastfeeding Support Groups

_____

_____

La Leche League International

www.lalecheleague.org

La Leche League International (LLLI) is a breastfeeding promotion organization started by breastfeeding mothers in 1956 to help other mothers with breastfeeding. In 1964, it became an international organization and continues to work around the world. To find a local La Leche League group, go to the Web site, choose a country and state, and search for local LLLI groups.

_____

_____

Human Milk Banking Association of North America

www.hmbana.org

The Human Milk Banking Association of North America is the organization of the 10 human milk banks in the United States and the one milk bank in Canada. Donated human milk is accepted from screened donors, pooled and pasteurized (using Holder pasteurization), and frozen until needed. To find the nearest milk bank or donor station near you, go to the Web site.

_____

_____

Adopted from Breastfeeding Resources by Mary O'Connor, MD, MPH, FAAP.

REFUSING BOTTLE, PREFERRING TO NURSE (BABY, LATER)

Definition

Baby refuses to drink from bottle, and mother needs to be able to leave baby with other caregivers. Baby may wait for mom to return and may go 8 hours without liquids.

BACKGROUND

- Preference for breast and nursing time with mother.
- Can occur with delayed introduction of bottle beyond 4-week period.
- Mother must also be motivated to stay away long enough so baby will get hungry enough to try the bottle.

TRIAGE ASSESSMENT QUESTIONS

Home Care

○ Concern for refusing bottle in context of adequate hydration

HOME CARE ADVICE

❶ **Rest Assured:** Babies usually do not get dehydrated or lose weight in this refusal process. Continue monitoring wet diapers and if decreased in last 8 hours, resume nursing and try at another time.

❷ **Consider Nipple Confusion:** If planning to return to work or school before your baby is 6 months of age, it is best to try pumped milk in a bottle after 4 weeks of age when milk supply is established. Nipple confusion can occur in about 25% of babies if attempted before 1 month of age.

❸ **Round Up a Family Suspect:** At any age, you need a motivated caregiver to try to feed your baby in a quiet, dark room once you have left the building.

❹ **Try a Cup:** If infant is older than 6 months, try different nipples or a cup with a soft spout with pumped human milk.

❺ **Call Back If:** Advice not helping. See within 3 days in office (by appointment).

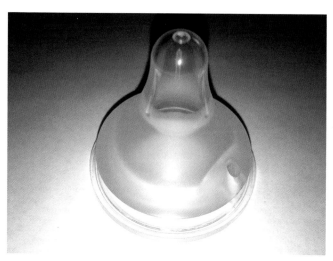

"Like Momma" soft nipple

SLEEPY NEWBORN (BABY, EARLY)

Definition

Some babies fall asleep at the breast or do not wake easily for feedings, which usually gets better after 6 to 8 weeks of age.

TRIAGE ASSESSMENT QUESTIONS

See Other Protocol

- Late Preterm Newborn on page 51

See Today Immediately

- Skipped or slept thought a feeding, is difficult to awaken, and has not been a sleepy baby since birth
  Reason: concern for systemic illness

See Within 3 Days in Office *(by Appointment)*

- Has poor latch and did not feed well in hospital
  Reason: evaluation for latch, possible nipple shield, and pumping plan for long-term mechanical milk expression

Home Care

- Sleepy on and off at the breast
- Nursing adequately and may or may not feed better with a bottle
- Day and night mix-up

HOME CARE ADVICE

❶ **Place Skin to Skin:** Placing your baby, wearing only a diaper, on your chest is a good strategy. It can help her get tuned in to feeding. It has been shown to help preterm newborns experience more stable respiratory and heart rates and temperature. Skin-to-skin time can help increase milk volume. It will help keep your baby awake as well while nursing.

❷ **Pump:** You will need to pump occasionally for the early weeks until your baby wakes more predictably.

❸ **Keep Baby on Task:** If your baby is feeding, trying to keep her awake at the breast is a challenge. Holding her hand up in the air or tickling her under the axilla or feet can help.

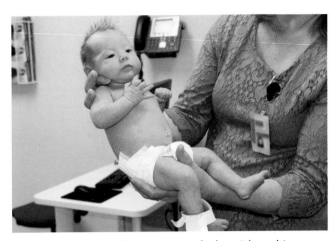
Suspending the baby in air may help with waking.

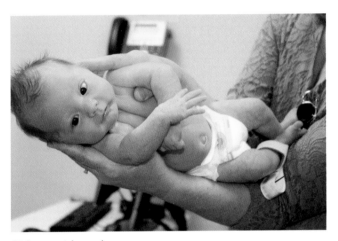
Side-to-side wake-up maneuver

❹ **Roll Side to Side or Change Diaper Between Breasts:** Gently rolling your baby side to side cradled in both forearms can be effective. Some babies wake up with diaper changes.

❺ **Switch Nursing:** Switching sides frequently (every 5 minutes, 4 times in total) during a nursing session can keep your baby awake and help with milk supply.

❻ **Keep Day Bright and Noisy and Night Quiet and Dark:** Have your baby sleep in the main area of the house where more noise and light is during the day, and make nighttime calm, quiet, and dark. For example, use a nightlight and minimize talking. This may take up to 2 weeks to fix.

❼ **Call Back If:** Advice not helping. See within 3 days in office (by appointment).

BACKGROUND INFORMATION

- Sleepiness is common in the first few weeks after birth in some full-term newborns.
- Sleepiness is more common in babies younger than 37 weeks. Late preterm newborns often have neurologic disorganization; latch may be poor, suck may be weak, newborn may not show feeding cues consistently, and newborn can go from hyperalert to in a very deep sleep, rapidly shutting down.

SORE NIPPLES (MOTHER)

Definition

- Sore, irritated nipples present with a wide range of descriptions, from mild discomfort with latching on to excruciating pain including related redness or cracking or scabbing.
- Occurs in about one-third of mothers.

TRIAGE ASSESSMENT QUESTIONS

See Other Protocol

- Appendix B: Quick Reference for Pain With Breastfeeding on page 109
- Breast Pain on page 6
- Tongue-tie on page 102
- Nursing With Pregnancy on page 85
- Overactive Letdown/Overabundant Milk Supply on page 86

See Today in Office (by Appointment)

- Lesions on nipple blister-like in appearance
- Any history of herpes
  Reason: herpes on nipples or breast is a contraindication for breastfeeding and, therefore, needs urgent testing and treatment

See Within 3 Days in Office (by Appointment)

- Painful latch
  Reason: should be evaluated; suspect improper latch or tongue-tie
- Increased redness
  Reason: suspect infection—any break in skin can cause infection; may need antibiotics and culture for methicillin-resistant Staphylococcus aureus
- Pink nipples, peeling skin, shooting pain, prone to yeast infections, received peripartum antibiotics
  Reason: suspect Candida infection even if baby does not have white plaques
- Blanching or color change of nipple (blue, white, or red)
- Sensitivity to cold or any similar symptoms of nipples in pregnancy
- Symptoms with vasoconstrictor medications, such as nicotine, caffeine, terbutaline, or theophylline
  Reason: suspect Raynaud disease; needs help to correct latch and possible nifedipine

Home Care

- Sores, cracks, or scabs on the nipple
- White-looking blebs (often described as "white dots")
- History of eczema and eczema lesions on breast
- New pregnancy causing nipple sensitivity in nursing mother
- Overabundant milk supply and baby may be pinching or clamping nipple to control flow

HOME CARE ADVICE

❶ **Pain Control:** May take ibuprofen (eg, Advil, Motrin); because of its anti-inflammatory properties, it is the best choice for pain.

❷ **Review of Latch Technique:** Promote proper latching by encouraging your baby to open her mouth wide by tickling her lips with your finger or nipple. Pull your baby close by supporting the back (rather than the back of the head) so that the chin dives into the breast and the nose is touching the breast at the nipple. Your baby can also be encouraged to latch on with some expressed milk. The nipple should be round when it goes into your baby's mouth, and you should make sure that it is not discolored, white, or pale when it comes out. Always break your baby's suction with your finger when she is coming off the breast.

❸ **Lanolin and Hydrogel/Soothies Pads for Cracks or Scabs:** Keep nipples covered with a medical-grade pure lanolin ointment and a hydrogel dressing, or Soothies Gel Pads, which will encourage any cracks to heal without scabbing or crusting. (These supplies can be found at Target and Babies"R"Us, respectively). To cool them, place on a clean plate in the refrigerator while nursing. Mini–ice packs can be made out of freezing 4" × 4" gauze in a resealable bag in the freezer. Tea bags, a former folklore remedy, are no longer recommended because the tannic acid in the tea is an astringent and can cause drying and cracking. Note: Washing lanolin off nipples is not needed. You may also see blood in the stool, but this is not harmful to your baby.

❹ **Rest Assured:** As a result of swallowed blood from cracked nipples, you may also see blood in the stool, but this is not harmful to your baby.

❺ **Blebs:** Blebs are thought to be a blocked pore (white dot) caused when milk seeps into the epidermis. Most blebs break on their own. Apply warm compresses, or try to break them open with a washcloth, tweezers, or a needle. If not successful, you should be seen to get lanced in the physician's office.

❻ **Eczema:** If you have known eczema, you may apply over-the-counter hydrocortisone cream. Wipe it off before the next nursing session.

❼ **Raynaud Disease:** Relief of vasospasm associated with the change in temperature that occurs when your baby breaks the latch can be helped with the following maneuvers:
- Press a flexed arm hard across the nipple/breast as soon as your baby is off the breast.
- Apply warm packs as soon as your baby comes off.

❽ **Clamping With Overactive Letdown:** Flow is forceful with letdowns during a feeding, and your baby may be clamping down on the nipple to try to control flow.
- Pump off the foremilk. To help decrease foremilk as well as volume that your baby may get at the start of feeds, pump off the foremilk (first 5 minutes). Label and save this milk for later; you may need to eventually mix it with other pumped milk.
- Offer only one breast per feed. Best to move to one-sided feedings: allow your baby to finish one side completely; only pump off the undrained side if needed for comfort purposes.
- Lean back with nursing because this gives baby better control over the flow.

❾ **Yeast Infection of the Nipples:** Nipple or areolar tissue may be flaky, red, itchy, and associated with a burning cessation. *All-purpose nipple ointment*, or APNO (mupirocin ointment, 2%; betamethasone ointment, 0.1%; and miconazole powder), is a popular approach to this infection, but individual tailored use of topical treatment is preferred. Systemic treatment with oral Diflucan and treatment of a baby with nystatin oral suspension or gentian violet is considered more effective.

❿ **Call Back If:** Advice not helping. See within 3 days in office (by appointment).

BACKGROUND INFORMATION

- This requires urgent assessment because it is the top reason mothers stop breastfeeding in the first 2 weeks postpartum.
- New mothers also give pain or discomfort as a reason to not breastfeed exclusively.
- Most mothers feel latch discomfort that subsides in the first minute if the baby has a wide, deep latch and coordinated suck.

Causes
- **Poor Latch:** Sore nipples may develop from a poor latch, disorganized sucking, or the baby not drawing enough of the areolar area into his mouth. The most common cause of sore nipples is improper positioning of the baby at the breast, resulting in improper latch.
- **Normal Discomfort:** Some mothers, even with a perfect latch, experience discomfort in the first few days as they "get used to breastfeeding." Vacuum suction to nipples every 2 hours is a new phenomenon for new mothers!
- **High Suckling Pressure:** Nipple blanching occurs from a "barracuda baby's" increased suckling pressure or from a baby latching and feeding on the nipple only.
- **Herpes:** Lesions on the mother's nipple or areola are a contraindication to nursing.
- *Candida* **(Yeast) Infection:** Intense, persistent nipple pain associated with burning or shooting. Often the nipple is pink tinged before the baby's mouth has white plaques.

- **Tongue-tie:** Short and tight lingular frenulum where the tongue is incapable of covering the lower gum and the baby is unable to create adequate sucking pressures because of restricted tongue elevation. This condition can cause discomfort and can appear as a heart-shaped end of the tongue that does not extend outward with crying.
- **Other Baby Anomalies:** High palate, torticollis, or mandibular asymmetry.
- **Blebs:** Shiny white bumps on tip of the nipple ("white dots") that cause pinpoint pain when the baby feeds. Blebs are thought to be blocked pores caused when milk seeps into the epidermis. When it completely blocks the flow of milk, stasis and plugged ducts can occur.
- **Eczema of the Nipple:** Red, dry, flaking rash.
- **Raynaud Vasospasm of the Nipple:** Rare but treatable cause of nipple pain. Symptoms usually start in pregnancy with sensitivity to cold and stimulation. Fixing the latch is still first-line management for this condition. After in-person evaluation, nifedipine can be prescribed for a trial 2-week period if vasospasm continues despite proper positioning and latching. Also, nifedipine can be trialed if chronic deep breast pain persists for 4 weeks or longer despite therapy with antifungals or antibacterials.
- **Clamping to Control Flow:** Pinching off or clenching of the nipple by the baby can occur to protect from forceful ejection reflex with overabundant milk supply or overactive letdown.

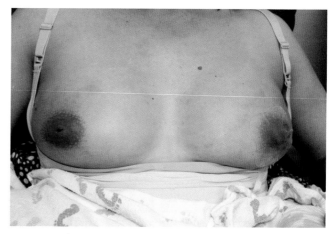

Sore nipple wound on right breast and nipple with gel pad covering on left breast

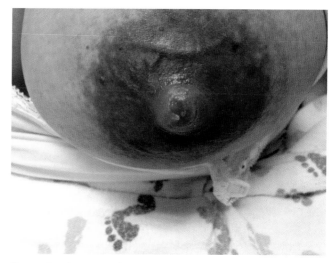

Sore nipple wound

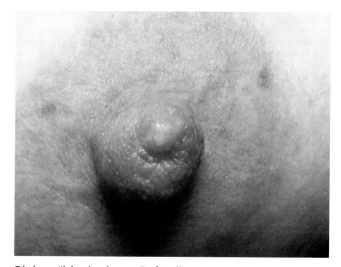

Bleb or "blocked pore" of milk

SPITTING UP (REFLUX) (BABY, EARLY)

Definition
- The effortless spitting up (reflux) of 1 or 2 mouthfuls of breast milk or formula
- Normal symptom in half of young infants
- **Excluded:** Vomiting (forceful throwing up of large amount)

TRIAGE ASSESSMENT QUESTIONS

Call EMS 911 Now
- Sounds like a life-threatening emergency to the triager

Go to ED Now
- Newborn < 4 weeks with fever 100.4° F (38.0° C) or higher rectally
  R/O: sepsis

Go to ED Now (or to Office With PCP Approval)
- Age 4 - 12 weeks with fever 100.4° F (38.0° C) or higher rectally
  R/O: sepsis
- Choked on milk and difficulty breathing persists
  R/O: aspiration pneumonia
- Choked on milk and turned bluish
  R/O: wake apnea due to aspirated milk
- Choked on milk and became limp
  R/O: hypotonia caused by hypoxia
- Newborn < 4 weeks starts to look or act abnormal in any way
  R/O: sepsis
- Child sounds very sick or weak to triager
  R/O: sepsis

Go to Office Now
- Contains blood
  (Note: have the caller bring in a sample of the blood for testing)
  R/O: reflux esophagitis
- Bile (green color) in the spit-up
  R/O: GI obstruction
- Pyloric stenosis suspected (age < 4 months and projectile vomiting 2 or more times)

- Taking reflux meds and severe crying/screaming that can't be consoled

See Today or Tomorrow in Office
- Caller wants child seen

See Within 3 Days in Office
- Chokes frequently on milk and mild
- Coughing illness persists > 3 weeks
  R/O: aspiration pneumonia
- Poor weight gain
  R/O: failure to thrive due to severe reflux
- Frequent, unexplained fussiness
  R/O: reflux esophagitis
- Caller wants to switch formulas
- Spitting up becoming WORSE (e.g., increased amount)
- Taking reflux meds and not helping
  R/O: eosinophilic esophagitis

See Within 2 Weeks in Office
- Not improved after using this care advice > 1 week
- Age > 12 months
  R/O: hiatal hernia; GER should be resolved

Home Care
- Normal reflux (spitting up) with no complications

HOME CARE ADVICE

1. **Reassurance and Education:**
   - It sounds like normal spitting up or reflux.
   - Reflux occurs in over 50% of infants.
   - Some simple measures can reduce the amount that's spit up.
   - Usually it doesn't cause any discomfort, crying, or complications.
   - Infants with normal reflux do not need any tests or medicines.

2. **Feed Smaller Amounts:**
   - Reason: Overfeeding or filling the stomach to capacity always makes spitting up worse.
   - Note: Skip this advice if age less than 1 month or not gaining weight well.
   - **Bottle-fed:** Give smaller amounts per feeding (1 ounce or 30 mL less than you have been).

- **Breastfed:** If you have a plentiful milk supply, try nursing on 1 side per feeding and pumping the other side. Alternate sides you start on. Keep the total feeding time to less than 20 minutes.

❸ **Longer Feeding Intervals:**
  - **Formula:** Wait at least 2½ hours between feedings.
  - **Breast Milk:** Wait at least 2 hours between feedings.
  (Reason: It takes that long for the stomach to empty itself. Don't add food to a full stomach.)

❹ **Loose Diapers:** Avoid tight diapers. It puts added pressure on the stomach. Don't put pressure on the abdomen or play vigorously with your child right after meals.

❺ **Vertical Position:**
  - After meals, try to hold your baby in the upright (vertical) position. Use a front pack, backpack, or swing for 30 to 60 minutes.
  - Reduce time in sitting position (e.g., infant seats).
  - After 6 months of age, a jumpy seat is helpful (the newer ones are stable).
  - Even during breast- or bottle-feedings, keep your baby's head higher than the stomach. Hold her at a slant.

❻ **Less Pacifier Time:**
  - Constant sucking on a pacifier can pump the stomach up with swallowed air.
  - So can sucking on a bottle with too small a nipple hole. If the formula doesn't drip out at a rate of 1 drop per second when held upside down, clean the nipple better or enlarge the hole.

❼ **Burping:**
  - Burping is less important than giving smaller feedings. You can burp your baby 2 or 3 times during each feeding.
  - Do it when he pauses and looks around. Don't interrupt his feeding rhythm to burp him.
  - Burp each time for less than a minute.
  - Stop even if no burp occurs. Some babies don't need to burp.

❽ **Expected Course:** Reflux improves with age. Many babies are better by 7 months of age, after learning to sit well.

❾ **Call Back If:**
  - It becomes vomiting.
  - Your baby doesn't improve with this approach.
  - Your child becomes worse.

❿ **Extra Advice—Rice Cereal and Thickened Feedings for Reflux Not Improved With Standard Treatment (Prefer Physician Approval):**
  - Thickened feedings mean adding cereal to formula until it is the consistency of a milk shake.
  - The correct mixture is usually 2 teaspoons (10 mL) of dry rice cereal per ounce (30 mL) of formula.
  - Breastfed babies can be offered rice cereal mixed with breast milk.

⓫ **Extra Advice—Sleeping Position:**
  - Babies who spit up can sleep on the back (the recommended position for normal infants).
  - When awake and supervised, however, the prone (tummy-down) position is better for protecting the lower esophagus.

⓬ **Extra Advice—Acid-Blocking Medicines:**
  - Medicines that block acid production are not helpful for normal reflux.
  - These medicines can have side effects.
  - They also do not help normal crying or colic.

BACKGROUND INFORMATION

Symptoms
- Smaller amounts often occur with burping ("wet burps").
- Larger amounts can occur after overfeeding or severe reflux.
- Usually seen during or shortly after feedings.
- Occurs mainly in children under 1 year of age and begins in the first weeks of life.
- Caution: Normal reflux does not cause any crying.

Complications
- These complications occur in less than 1% of infants:
  - Choking on spit-up milk.
  - Heartburn from acid on lower esophagus (reflux esophagitis). Infants with reflux esophagitis cry numerous times per day and act very unhappy when they are not crying. They are in almost constant discomfort.
  - Poor weight gain.

Spitting Up Severity Scale

- **Normal:** Spitting up small volumes after less than half the feeds.
- **Mild:** Spitting up small volumes after most feeds.
- **Moderate:** Spitting up larger volumes (half the feed) but good weight gain.
- **Severe:** Spitting up larger volumes (half the feed) and poor weight gain.

Cause

- Poor closure of the valve at the upper end of the stomach.
- Main Trigger: Overfeeding of formula or breast milk.
- More than half of all infants have occasional spitting up ("happy spitters").

Reflux Versus Vomiting: How to Tell

- **Parent Reports:** It's hard for parents to distinguish normal spitting up from vomiting. Most of what parents call vomiting is actually spitting up. This is an important distinction. While reflux is benign, vomiting in babies has a serious etiology until proven otherwise (such as pyloric stenosis). The following tips may help:
- **Reflux:** The following suggest reflux (spitting up): infant previously diagnosed with reflux, onset early in life (85% by 7 days of life), present for several days or weeks, no effort, no discomfort during reflux, no diarrhea, hungry, looks well, and acts happy.
- **Vomiting:** The following suggest vomiting: uncomfortable during vomiting, new symptom starting today or yesterday, sudden onset, associated diarrhea or fever, projectile or forceful vomiting, vomiting comes out the nose, contains bile, or child looks or acts sick.
- **Volume:** Vomiting usually brings up a large volume of stomach contents. The vomiting is usually forceful or projectile and the child is uncomfortable. Spitting up (reflux) usually involves smaller amounts.
- However, with gastroesophageal reflux, the volume of reflux can fluctuate. The amount can become larger if the child is wearing a tight diaper, is held in the horizontal position, or the size of the feeding was particularly large. Therefore, the amount is not that helpful to distinguishing between these 2 entities. With reflux, if the large amount comes out forcefully, the baby has changed to vomiting and may also have pyloric stenosis.

Pyloric Stenosis: How to Recognize

- **Definition:** Stomach outlet obstruction (narrowing) caused by hypertrophy of the pylorus muscle.
- **Symptoms:** The main symptom is projectile vomiting (the milk shoots out of the mouth). Other symptoms include vomit is not bilious, hungry after vomiting ("hungry vomiter," unlike babies with gastritis), and weight loss.
- **Peak Age:** 2 to 8 weeks. Rare after 3 months. More common in firstborn males.
- **Diagnostic Test:** Ultrasound.
- **Treatment:** Surgery.

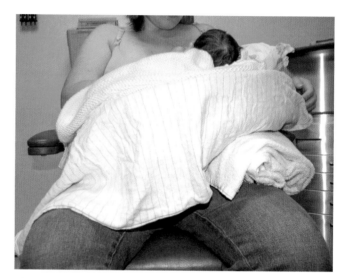

Slanted feeding position even while nursing

SUBSTANCES OF ABUSE (ILLICIT DRUGS) (MOTHER)

Definition

- **The effortless spitting up (reflux) of 1 or 2 mouthfuls of breast milk or formula**
- **Normal symptom in half of young infants**
- **Excluded:** Vomiting (forceful throwing up of large amount)

TRIAGE ASSESSMENT QUESTIONS

Go to ED Now

- ● Baby exposed to any illicit drugs
- ● Any symptoms of irritability or sedation in baby
  Reason: "the lack of pharmacokinetic data for most drugs of abuse in recently postpartum women precludes the establishment of a 'safe' interval after use when breastfeeding can be reestablished for individual drugs of abuse" (Academy of Breastfeeding Medicine protocol); may need to report to social services if mother does not adhere to emergent evaluation

See Other Protocol

- ● Maternal Medications (Advice Only) (psychotropic medications) on page 67
- ● Alcohol Use on page 1
- ● Marijuana Use on page 61
- ● Maternal Smoking, Vaping, and Cessation Strategies on page 73

BACKGROUND INFORMATION

- More than 5% of pregnant women 15 to 44 years of age reported use of illicit drugs in the past month, according to the 2016 National Survey on Drug Use and Health.
- Entering treatment program prior to delivery is recommended if planning to breastfeed. Because mothers with a history of drug abuse are at high risk of relapse, there is concern that they may not necessarily stay clean when breastfeeding. Being in an active treatment program will help mothers maintain abstinence and help ensure the safety of their baby.

- Cocaine, amphetamines, heroin, and phencyclidine are detected in human milk in high concentrations and, therefore, can pass quickly to the baby.
- Marijuana and metabolites are viewed as less severe drugs of abuse but can have dangerous contaminants. Marijuana has a long half-life, but current evidence cannot determine safe time after exposure to start breastfeeding.
- Brain cell development is taking place in the first months after birth, and long-term developmental effects of illicit drugs through human milk are unknown.
- Methadone and buprenorphine are used to treat mothers with opioid addiction and are considered safe in breastfeeding. For mothers in active treatment who are being followed with routine urine toxicology testing, breastfeeding can be encouraged if screening results are negative. If there are concerns that mother is not adherent to treatment or is using illicit substances, breastfeeding is not considered a safe option.
- Babies who are exposed to methadone during pregnancy are at HIGH RISK of experiencing neonatal abstinence syndrome, or withdrawal from the methadone. Babies may experience less neonatal abstinence syndrome when breastfeeding because of the small amounts of methadone delivered in human milk.
- Mothers with a history of substance abuse often have comorbid issues of mental illness, HIV, hepatitis, smoking, and alcohol. Determination of maternal use as casual/occasional versus habitual is difficult.

TANDEM NURSING (SPECIAL CIRCUMSTANCES)

Definition

Nursing 2 children of different ages simultaneously

TRIAGE ASSESSMENT QUESTIONS

See Other Protocol

● Overactive Letdown/Overabundant Milk Supply on page 86

● Breast Pain (for engorgement) on page 6

Home Care

○ Concerns about enough milk for both

○ Overabundant milk supply

○ Ongoing engorgement

Note: triage practitioner should be sure to assess 8 key breastfeeding questions about newborn

HOME CARE ADVICE

❶ **Feeding Order:** Feed your youngest baby first; colostrum should go to newborn first. Allow older child to finish as needed. There will be enough milk for 2.

❷ **Positioning:** May be stressful to successfully position and nurse 2 just as with breastfeeding multiples. An older toddler usually is flexible and even creative in this regard.

❸ **Infectious Exposure:** No need to wash breasts or nipples between children, but thorough hand-washing is always a good practice when an older child is around a newborn.

❹ **Engorgement:** It can be more severe when tandem nursing; often a toddler can help relieve it more effectively than a newborn can.

❺ **Overabundant Supply:** Because this is a subsequent child and more breast stimulation and emptying is occurring, it is not usual to have an overabundant milk supply. This may pose difficulties for your newborn.

❻ **Maternal Self-care:** Tandem nursing can be psychologically demanding; make sure to get rest, nourishment, and drinks to satisfy thirst.

❼ **Call Back If:** Advice not helping. See within 3 days in office (by appointment).

BACKGROUND INFORMATION

- Situation most often occurs when a newborn arrives into the family and the toddler is still nursing.
- If the mother has a preterm newborn or another reason for compromised milk supply, the tandem nursing child can help stimulate milk supply.
- Mothers often want to avoid abrupt weaning because nursing is a comfort for the older child. At the same time, birth of a new baby can be a stressor for the older child.

Note: Kangaroo mothers have 2 different teats in their pouches, one for the older joey and one for the newborn; they put out milk of appropriate maturity for each offspring. Humans do not have that capacity. A human mother's milk will transition to the type appropriate for her newborn rather than for the other child.

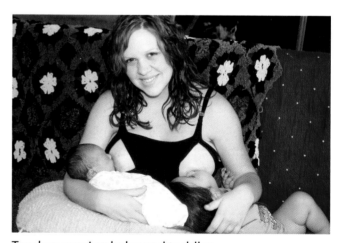

Tandem nursing baby and toddler

TASTE CHANGE OF HUMAN MILK (BABY, EARLY)

Definition

- Soapy, metallic, or fishy smell to thawed frozen or refrigerated milk.
- Taste change can also be caused by new or different food or medication or prolonged exercise and lactic acid buildup.

TRIAGE ASSESSMENT QUESTIONS

See Other Protocol

- Milk Storage and Return to Work/School on page 75
- Maternal Ingestion of Foods and Herbs (Advice Only) on page 66
- Nursing With Pregnancy on page 85

Home Care

- Milk that smells or tastes soapy, metallic, or fishy
  R/O lipase
- Mother who tried new foods, medications, or strenuous exercise
  R/O other causes
- Sour and lumpy, like spoiled bovine milk in carton
  R/O contaminated milk

HOME CARE ADVICE

❶ **Rest Assured:** If baby takes it, do not worry.

❷ **Refusal May Be Because of Taste:** Try mixing it 1:1 with fresh milk. Scalding the milk prior to storing destroys the lipase. It should be cooled and frozen as soon as possible after scalding.

❸ **Suspect Other Cause:** Consider changing diet or medication or making adjustments in exercise.

❹ **Check if Contaminated Human Milk:** Unfortunately, this milk should be discarded.

BACKGROUND INFORMATION

- Lipase enzyme breaks down fat in milk; occurs more readily at colder temperatures. Some women produce more lipase than others.
- Human milk also takes on taste of whatever a mother eats, including medications (eg, if mother eats garlic, milk will taste like garlic). Later this increases the baby's acceptance of solids.
- After prolonged or strenuous exercise, a mother's milk can taste sour because of lactic acid buildup.

TONGUE-TIE (BABY, EARLY)

Definition

- Anatomic abnormality involving short, tight lingular frenulum where the tongue is functionally incapable of covering the lower gum and is often limited in tongue elevation, lateralization, and cupping.
- This condition can appear as a heart-shaped end of the tongue, most notably seen when the baby attempts to extend tongue outward with licking lips or crying.

TRIAGE ASSESSMENT QUESTIONS

See Other Protocol

- Sore Nipples on page 93
- Clicking or Noisy Nursing on page 14
- Overactive Letdown/Overabundant Milk Supply on page 86

See Within 3 Days in Office (by Appointment)

- Tongue with notch or heart shaped
- Tongue that does not protrude easily and retracts with crying or moves side to side with gum massage
- Painful latch for mother
- Baby who comes off breast frequently
- Baby who makes noises with nursing
- Choking or crying with feedings
  R/O overactive letdown
- Maternal frustration with inefficient nursing
  Reason: suspect tongue-tie; lactation assistance can be useful and may obviate surgical intervention

HOME CARE ADVICE

Pumping Until Evaluation Is Best: If your baby is frustrated with feedings or you are having nipple pain, you should pump instead until referral can be made for latch evaluation or frenectomy.

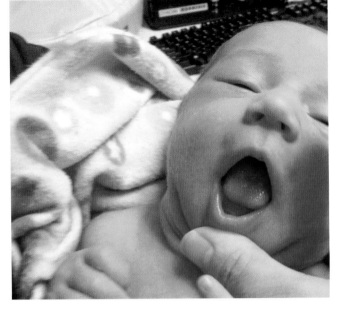

Tongue does not protrude beyond the baby's gumline. Note indentation at tip of tongue.

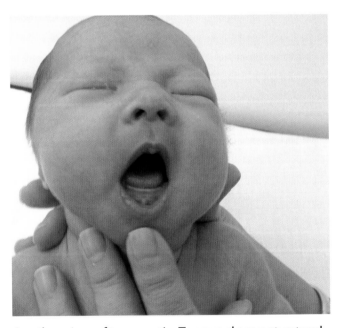

Another view of tongue-tie. Tongue does not extend beyond the gums, causing maternal pain and ineffective milk transfer.

BACKGROUND INFORMATION

- Of babies, 0.02% to 10.7% have congenital ankyloglossia (ie, tongue-tie being present at birth).
- Condition can be familial.
- Fifty percent of babies with tongue-tie will not have breastfeeding difficulty.
- There is some concern that this is a condition is a fad driven by practitioners who are making money from this procedure, which is not generally covered by insurance providers.
- Controversy exists on significance of this condition and when clipping is indicated. Recent systematic reviews on the topic suggested more rigorous research is needed.
- Sometimes clipping is needed to reduce pain in the mother or for improved milk transfer.
- Can be performed by pediatrician or family physician (if trained in frenotomy/frenectomy), otolaryngologist, or dentist. Usually procedure is performed with sucrose analgesia alone (ie, without anesthesia). The baby can usually nurse immediately afterward.
- Unfortunately, some infants can have issues after laser treatment with scarring.
- Although many believe that it can be associated with later speech difficulties, little evidence supports this. If tongue-tie is not causing breastfeeding issues, the American Speech-Language-Hearing Association recommends waiting until age 4 years for assessment. As the child grows, the lingual frenulum recedes, stretches, and may even rupture, so initial restrictions of lingual movement are diminished.

VITAMIN D, IRON, AND ZINC SUPPLEMENTATION (BABY, EARLY)

GENERAL CONSIDERATIONS

Vitamin D

- Lack of intake or sun exposure leads to vitamin D deficiency and can cause growth delay.
- Because of the success of public health awareness of skin cancer risk, the avoidance of sun exposure has resulted in an increase in rickets in some babies (even in sunny areas of the United States).
- In addition, vitamin D deficiency is being linked to many other illnesses in adults and children (eg, poor growth).
- The American Academy of Pediatrics now recommends that all babies receive 400 IU of vitamin D per day starting soon after birth. Exclusively breastfed babies should receive vitamin D in the form of an oral supplement until they are consuming at least 32 ounces of vitamin D–fortified milk (formula if younger than 1 year, carton/jug milk if older than 1 year).
- Mothers who are receiving 6,400 IU of vitamin D as a supplement do not need to supplement their babies.
- Previously, 20 minutes of sun twice a week that involved face and full arms was recommended for babies. However, this is no longer recommended because of the baby's risk of sunburn and lifetime risk of skin cancer. Also, babies who are darker skinned do not absorb as much sunlight and are, therefore, at higher risk of rickets if no vitamin D supplementation is given.
- One study indicates that only 5% to 10% of pediatricians self-report adherence to these recommendations.

Iron

- Stores that the baby received in utero from mother start to decrease at 4 to 6 months of age. In a 2010 clinical report, the American Academy of Pediatrics recommends giving breastfed infants at 4 months of age 1 mg/kg/d of a liquid iron supplement until solid foods, such as meats or iron-fortified cereals, are introduced at 6 months of age.

Zinc

- Zinc deficiency can be associated with growth failure and increased susceptibility to infections.

Supplementation, beyond the usual diet, to the breastfeeding mother or breastfed infant is not routinely recommended.

TRIAGE ASSESSMENT QUESTIONS

Home Care

○ Exclusively breastfeeding and wonder whether vitamin D, zinc, or iron is necessary

○ Spitting up or refusal of vitamin D or multivitamin preparation

HOME CARE ADVICE

❶ **Exclusively Breastfed Babies Need Vitamin D:** "Exclusively breastfed" means no liquids other than water or medication besides human milk. If mixed feeding, your baby needs to consume a minimum of 32 ounces of vitamin D–fortified milk.

❷ **May Need Iron:** Babies' iron stores start to diminish as stores from their mothers decrease at 4 to 6 months of age. Babies can have their hemoglobin levels checked if there are any growth concerns.

❸ **Dosing and Types of Preparations:** All are available over the counter and do not require a prescription.
- **Multivitamin Preparation With Vitamin D 400 IU/mL Includes Iron (eg, D-Vi-Sol, Poly-Vi-Sol):** Give your baby 1 mL (1 dropperful) per day.
- **Carlson Kid's Drops:** Single-drop preparation has 400 IU per drop, is tasteless, and can be applied to your nipple immediately prior to nursing.

❹ **Spitting-up Preparation:** If frequent spitting up of dose is noted (not uncommon with the multivitamin preparation due to metallic taste), you can try to split the dose into several doses, trickling it in through the side of the mouth while your baby is nursing, or an alternative preparation.

❺ **Continue Avoiding Sun Exposure:** Protect your baby's skin with a hat, long-sleeved clothes, and an umbrella or a stroller awning. Apply sunscreen (30 SPF) prior to going outside to infants older than 6 months.

WEANING (BABY, LATER)

Definition
- **Mother-Led Weaning:** Mother interested in trying to stop breastfeeding.
- **Child-Led Weaning:** Normal periods of distraction in baby/toddler when going through developmental milestones can be opportunities for weaning.
- **Early Weaning (Earlier Than 1 Year):** Necessary for other reasons (eg, difficult work or school environment, family stress, baby illness or death).

TRIAGE ASSESSMENT QUESTIONS

See Other Protocol
- Nursing Strike or Refusal on page 84
- Milk Storage and Return to Work/School on page 75

Home Care
- ○ Weaning is desired and timing not premature (ie, later than 1 year)

HOME CARE ADVICE

❶ Reassurance: Be patient. Weaning is a challenging process for most mother-child pairs.

❷ Weaning Younger Than 1 Year
- This may be a nursing strike or another kind of phase, so best to pump until your baby resumes nursing again.
- If there is an abrupt need to wean, you may need to express small amounts of milk for comfort; use ice packs and ibuprofen if in pain. A cup of sage tea or a single dose of pseudoephedrine are home remedies that may help. Cabergoline is a newer medication that may be prescribed by your physician in certain circumstances.

❸ Child-Led Weaning Later Than 1 Year: Look for windows of weaning. Anticipate these opportunities for weaning when your infant/toddler may have a distracted phase, especially in times of developmental changes.

❹ Mother-Led Weaning Later Than 1 Year
- Go slow. Drop a feeding every few days. This will allow for your breasts to adjust and result in less pain or engorgement.
- Offer sippy cup. In place of a nursing session, offer a sippy cup with water or milk.
- Keep busy. For example, go for walks outside in stroller, or go on outings to a zoo or museum.
- Wear restricted clothing. Keeping covered up helps prevent access to breasts (ie, more covering than just a camisole top).
- Take care of nighttime weaning first. Try to take care of eliminating nighttime feedings first and then taper daytime feeds. May need to make changes about where your toddler sleeps and encourage a bedtime blanket or another kind of cuddly object for comfort.

❺ Recommended Reading: See References on page 111.

❻ Mother May Need an Extended Outing: Occasionally, resistant children require that the mother stay away for a more extended period.

❼ Call Back If: Advice not helping. See within 3 days in office (by appointment).

BACKGROUND INFORMATION
- Premature weaning (before 1 year of age or so) can be normal periods of distraction in infant with developmental milestones that are misinterpreted as infant's desire to wean.
- Prolonged nursing strike is misinterpreted as infant's desire to wean.

APPENDIX A
Breastfeeding Touchpoints for Overcoming Obstacles to Exclusivity

Breastfeeding Touchpoint	Parental Concern	Main Obstacles	Provider Advice
Prenatal	"I want to breastfeed, but since I am going to work, I need to be able to give formula too."	• Lack of information about combining breastfeeding and working • Lack of information about milk expression	• Strongly encourage attendance at a prenatal breastfeeding class (deserves equal time to birthing class education). • Consider a longer maternity leave, if possible. • Prepare to simplify life during the transition to parenting.
	"My husband and other family members will want to help feed the baby. Won't they feel excluded if I only breastfeed?"	• Family members wanting to feed the baby	• Enlist father's help in supporting his nursing partner. • Fathers can interact with their infant by holding baby skin-to-skin or taking baby out while mother sleeps. • After breastfeeding is well established, others can feed expressed milk by bottle.
	"I want to do combination feeding, or Los Dos."	• Desire for "the best of both worlds" by combination feeding • Lack of knowledge about the importance of frequent and exclusive breastfeeding during the early postpartum weeks for establishing mother's milk supply	• "Puro pecho," or only mother's own milk, provides greater health benefits and helps maintain an abundant milk supply. • If eligible, enrollment in WIC offers breastfeeding mothers a substantial food package, counseling, breast pumps, and peer counselors.
Birth	"My friend says it is a good idea to ask the nurses to care for my baby at night, so I can get some sleep."	• Unrealistic expectations for the postbirth hospital stay • Lack of prenatal education • Frequent interruptions and excessive visitors deplete new mothers. • Increased risk of formula supplements for nighttime births from 9 PM to 6 AM	• Promote immediate skin-to-skin contact after birth to facilitate initiation of breastfeeding within the first hour. • Teach mother to interpret her infant's feeding cues and breastfeed as often as baby wants. Advocate for no routine formula use in the system of care. • Advise mother to request help in the hospital with breastfeeding to promote task mastery. • Encourage continuous rooming-in, where mother can practice being with her baby in a controlled setting and learn to latch baby comfortably and effectively.
	"The yellow milk does not look like much. A little formula won't hurt, will it?"	• Belief that the small amount of colostrum is insufficient until "milk comes in"	• Explain the potency and adequacy of colostrum and the rapid increase in milk production from 36 to 96 h.
3–5 d	"Now that we are home, the baby seems to be feeding every hour. She or he doesn't seem satisfied."	• Lack of knowledge about normal frequency of feedings for breastfed newborns • Infants typically begin feeding more frequently the second night after birth, when baby is at home. • Concern about whether the infant is getting enough milk, due to mother's inability to see what the infant takes at the breast • Sleepy infant	• Explain that 8–12 feedings in 24 h are typical and necessary to establish an abundant milk supply. • Provide a hand-pump, or teach hand expression, so mother can see that she has milk. • Explain normal infant elimination patterns once mother's milk comes in (3–5 voids and 3–4 stools per day by 3–5 d; onset of yellow, seedy milk stools by 4–5 d). • Perform infant test weights (before and after feeding) to reassure mother about baby's milk intake at a feeding. • Teach mother the difference between infant "flutter sucking" or "nibbling" that results in only a trickle of milk at breast versus "drinking" milk, with active sucking and regular swallowing. • Tickling under axilla or holding hand up can help keep baby on task at breast. Or, compressing the breast when the baby stops slow, deep sucking can deliver a spray of milk to entice him or her to start drinking again. • Anticipate infant appetite spurt at about 10–14 d of age.
	"My nipples are sore and cracked. Can I take a break and give my baby a little formula?"	• Sore nipples usually are attributable to incorrect latch-on technique and are a common reason that mothers discontinue breastfeeding early or start supplements.	• Observe a nursing session to evaluate latch. Consider referring mother to a lactation consultant for one-on-one assistance with latch.
2 wk	"My breasts do not feel very full anymore. I'm afraid my milk went away."	• As postpartum breast engorgement resolves, and the breasts adjust to making and releasing milk, mothers may perceive they have insufficient milk.	• Expect infant to be above birth weight by 10–14 d, and reassure mother about infant's rate of weight gain since the 3–5-d visit. • Although mother's breasts are less swollen than during postpartum engorgement, they should feel fuller before feedings and softer afterward.
	"How can I know my baby is getting enough?"	• The 10–14-d appetite spurt can cause mother to doubt the adequacy of her milk supply.	• Consider performing test weights (before and after feeding) to reassure mother about her infant's intake. • Anticipate another appetite spurt at about 3 wk of age.

(continued on next page)

APPENDIX A
Breastfeeding Touchpoints for Overcoming Obstacles to Exclusivity

Breastfeeding Touchpoint	Parental Concern	Main Obstacles	Provider Advice
1 mo	"My baby is crying a lot, and I am tired and need sleep."	• Normal infant crying peaks at about 6 wk (3–5 h in 24 h). • Mother may attribute infant crying to hunger or an adverse reaction to her milk.	• Congratulate mother on a full month of breastfeeding! • If infant has gained weight appropriately, reassure mother about the adequacy of her milk supply. • Offer coping strategies for infant crying, including holding baby skin-to-skin; 5 Ss (however, swaddling with hands up near head to help assess feeding cues); use of infant carrier; stroller or car ride; Period of PURPLE Crying.
	"Nothing seems to calm her/him except the bottle."	• If infant drinks milk from a bottle that is offered, mother may assume infant is not satisfied by breastfeeding.	• Explain that infant sucking is reflexive, and drinking from an offered bottle doesn't always mean that the baby was hungry. Baby "can't scream and suck at the same time," so the bottle may appear to calm baby, just as a pacifier might. • If mom desires to offer a bottle, use expressed milk as the supplement. • Forewarn mother about cluster feeds (late afternoon/evening) and upcoming appetite spurts, occurring about 6 wk and 3 mo.
2 mo	"My mother said that, if I give rice cereal in a bottle before bedtime, the baby may sleep longer at night."	• Parental sleep deprivation • Mother may already have returned to work, which often increases fatigue and leads to a decrease in milk supply.	• Explain the lack of evidence that rice cereal or other solid foods increase infant sleep. • Remind mother that adding complementary foods is a project and increases workload for parents. • Reinforce the benefits of exclusive breastfeeding for maternal-infant health and mother's milk supply.
	"I am going back to work, and am worried that I do not have enough frozen stores of milk. Are there any herbs I can take to keep my milk supply strong?"	• Lack of knowledge about the principles of milk production and unrealistic beliefs about the efficacy of galactogogues	• Enlist help from others, including support for returning to work. • Explain that there is no "magic pill" or special tea to increase mother's milk supply. The key to ongoing milk production is frequent, effective milk removal (every 3–4 h). • Caution mother to avoid going long intervals without draining her breasts.
4 mo	"My baby seems to only eat for a few minutes, and when I try to put her/him back to the breast, she/he refuses."	• Misinterpretation of infant's efficiency in nursing causes concern about infant milk intake.	• Explain that infants become more efficient at breastfeeding, and by 3 mo, they may drain the breast in 4–7 min. • Reinforce continuing to delay the introduction of solid foods.
	"My baby seems more interested in everything around him/her than in nursing at the breast."	• Normal infant distractibility causes mother to believe her infant is self-weaning.	• Explain that distractibility is a normal developmental behavior at this age, and that short, efficient feeds are common. • Nurse in a quiet, darkened room.
6 mo	"My baby is drooling and rubbing on her/his gums all the time. I do not think that I can continue to breastfeed because my baby might bite me."	• Common myth that a mother needs to wean when her baby gets teeth to avoid being bitten while breastfeeding	• Congratulate mother on 6 mo of exclusive breastfeeding! • Explain that infants cannot bite and actively breastfeed at the same time. Biting tends to occur if the breast is offered when the infant is not interested or at the end of the feeding. • If the infant bites, say "No biting," touch the infant's lips, set the baby down, and briefly leave the room.
	"My baby has refused to breastfeed for almost a whole day now. Is she/he ready to wean?"	• Misinterpretation of sudden breastfeeding refusal ("Nursing Strike") to mean that a baby is self-weaning.	• Explain that some babies may suddenly refuse the breast between 4 and 7 mo of age for no apparent reason. • Common causes include an upper respiratory infection, ear infection, teething, regular exposure to bottlefeeding, use of a new soap/perfume, maternal stress, or a decrease in milk supply. • Because many babies will nurse while asleep, try offering the breast when the baby is drowsy or asleep. • Regularly express milk if the baby won't nurse, and feed the pumped milk until the infant resumes breastfeeding.

Courtesy of M. Bunik, MD, Aurora, CO.

APPENDIX B
Quick Reference for Pain With Breastfeeding

Inquiry	Cause of Pain	Recommendation
• Lips tucked under—"grandpa lips"? • Not opening wide enough and getting only nipple in mouth?	Poor latch	• Pull out lips. • Wait for wide-open mouth; may need to get to baby before too awake and hungry to increase cooperation.
• Early days' discomfort from baby's vacuum suction? • Any blanching?	Discomfort in first weeks vs high suckling pressure	• Lanolin • Deep breathing • Review of good latch
Blister-like lesions on breast?	Herpes	Avoid nursing on affected side.
• Pink-tinged nipples? • Itching? • Shooting pain in breast?	*Candida* infection	Simultaneous antifungal treatment of mother and baby (APNO not adequate)
• Does baby's tongue extend beyond gums? • Does baby's tongue move up and sideways when you rub the gums?	Tongue-tie, other mouth abnormalities	If any suspicion, get a formal evaluation. (Author's experience is that currently tongue-tie is a popular overdiagnosis.)
Shiny white dot on tip of nipple?	Bleb	Opening up with sterile needle, high rate of reoccurrence
• Dry, flaky rash? • History of allergies or eczema?	Eczema or irritant dermatitis	• OTC hydrocortisone and if no improvement may need more potent version by prescription • May have allergy to lanolin, detergents/bleach, soaps
• Sensitivity of nipples to cold or stimulation? • Color change of nipple after nursing?	Vasospasm of nipple/ Raynaud disease	Needs evaluation, will likely need prescription for nifedipine
• Plentiful milk supply? • Baby pulls off with squirts of milk a few minutes into a nursing session? • Blanching of the nipple?	Clamping down due to oversupply	Lean back with nursing because it affords baby better control of fast flow.
• Soreness beyond the nipple? • Area of redness of breast? • Fever?	Mastitis	Needs evaluation, will likely need antibiotics

Abbreviations: APNO, all-purpose nipple ointment; OTC, over-the-counter.

References for All Protocols

Alcohol Use

1. Hale TW, Berens P. *Clinical Therapy in Breastfeeding Patients*. 3rd ed. Amarillo, TX: Hale; 2011
2. Ho E, Collantes A, Kapur BM, Moretti M, Koren G. Alcohol and breast feeding: calculation of time to zero level in milk. *Biol Neonate*. 2001;80(3):219–222
3. Lawrence RA, Lawrence RM. *Breastfeeding: A Guide for the Medical Profession*. 8th ed. Philadelphia, PA: Elsevier; 2016
4. Texas Tech University Health Sciences Center. InfantRisk Center. http://www.infantrisk.com. Accessed March 29, 2018
5. Wilson J, Tay RY, McCormack C, et al. Alcohol consumption by breastfeeding mothers: frequency, correlates and infant outcomes. *Drug Alcohol Rev*. 2017;36(5):667–676

Allergy

1. Academy of Breastfeeding Medicine. ABM clinical protocol #24: allergic proctocolitis in the exclusively breastfed infant. *Breastfeed Med*. 2011;6(6):435–440
2. American Academy of Pediatrics. *New Mother's Guide to Breastfeeding*. Meek JY, ed. 3rd ed. New York, NY: Bantam Books; 2017
3. Greer FR, Sicherer SH, Burks AW; American Academy of Pediatrics Committee on Nutrition, Section on Allergy and Immunology. Effects of early nutritional interventions on the development of atopic disease in infants and children: the role of maternal dietary restriction, breastfeeding, timing of introduction of complementary foods, and hydrolyzed formulas. *Pediatrics*. 2008;121(1):183–191
4. Lawrence RA, Lawrence RM. *Breastfeeding: A Guide for the Medical Profession*. 8th ed. Philadelphia, PA: Elsevier; 2016
5. Rowe J, Kusel M, Holt BJ, et al. Prenatal versus postnatal sensitization to environmental allergens in a high-risk birth cohort. *J Allergy Clin Immunol*. 2007;119(5):1164–1173

Biting Breast, Onset at 6 Months

1. American Academy of Pediatrics. *New Mother's Guide to Breastfeeding*. Meek JY, ed. 3rd ed. New York, NY: Bantam Books; 2017
2. Neifert M. *Great Expectations: The Essential Guide to Breastfeeding*. New York, NY: Sterling Publishing; 2009

Breast Mass

1. Lawrence RA, Lawrence RM. *Breastfeeding: A Guide for the Medical Profession*. 8th ed. Philadelphia, PA: Elsevier; 2016
2. Lei X, Chen K, Zhu L, Song E, Su F, Li S. Treatments for idiopathic granulomatous mastitis: systematic review and meta-analysis. *Breastfeed Med*. 2017;12(7):415–421
3. Neifert M. *Great Expectations: The Essential Guide to Breastfeeding*. New York, NY: Sterling Publishing; 2009
4. Scott CR. Lecithin: it isn't just for plugged milk ducts and mastitis anymore. *Midwifery Today Int Midwife*. 2005;(76):26–27
5. Scott-Conner CE, Schorr SJ. The diagnosis and management of breast problems during pregnancy and lactation. *Am J Surg*. 1995; 170(4):401–405
6. Sheybani F, Sarvghad M, Naderi H, Gharib M. Treatment for and clinical characteristics of granulomatous mastitis. *Obstet Gynecol*. 2015;125(4):801–807

Breast Pain

1. Academy of Breastfeeding Medicine Protocol Committee. ABM clinical protocol #4: mastitis. Revision, May 2008. *Breastfeed Med*. 2008;3(3):177–180
2. Berens P; Academy of Breastfeeding Medicine Protocol Committee. ABM clinical protocol #20: engorgement. *Breastfeed Med*. 2009;4(2):111–113
3. Amir LH; Academy of Breastfeeding Medicine Protocol Committee. ABM clinical protocol #4: mastitis, revised March 2014. *Breastfeed Med*. 2014;9(5):239–243
4. Amir LH, Donath SM, Garland SM, et al. Does *Candida* and/or *Staphylococcus* play a role in nipple and breast pain in lactation? A cohort study in Melbourne, Australia. *BMJ Open*. 2013;3(3)
5. Barrett ME, Heller MM, Stone HF, Murase JE. Dermatoses of the breast in lactation. *Dermatol Ther*. 2013;26(4):331–336
6. Barrett ME, Heller MM, Stone HF, Murase JE. Raynaud phenomenon of the nipple in breastfeeding mothers: an underdiagnosed cause of nipple pain. *JAMA Dermatol*. 2013;149(3):300–306
7. Cota-Robles S, Pedersen L, LeCroy CW. Challenges to breastfeeding initiation and duration for teen mothers. *MCN Am J Matern Child Nurs*. 2017;42(3):173–178
8. Eglash A, Plane MB, Mundt M. History, physical and laboratory findings, and clinical outcomes of lactating women treated with antibiotics for chronic breast and/or nipple pain. *J Hum Lact*. 2006;22(4):429–433
9. Gateley CA, Miers M, Mansel RE, Hughes LE. Drug treatments for mastalgia: 17 years experience in the Cardiff Mastalgia Clinic. *J R Soc Med*. 1992;85(1):12–15
10. Jamali FR, Ricci A Jr, Deckers PJ. Paget's disease of the nipple-areola complex. *Surg Clin North Am*. 1996;76(2):365–381
11. Jiménez E, Arroyo R, Cárdenas N, et al. Mammary candidiasis: a medical condition without scientific evidence? *PLoS One*. 2017;12(7):e0181071
12. Lawrence RA, Lawrence RM. *Breastfeeding: A Guide for the Medical Profession*. 8th ed. Philadelphia, PA: Elsevier; 2016
13. Mangesi L, Dowswell T. Treatments for breast engorgement during lactation. *Cochrane Database Syst Rev*. 2010;(9):CD006946
14. Neifert M. *Great Expectations: The Essential Guide to Breastfeeding*. New York, NY: Sterling Publishing; 2009
15. Scott CR. Lecithin: it isn't just for plugged milk ducts and mastitis anymore. *Midwifery Today Int Midwife*. 2005;(76):26–27
16. Wong BB, Chan YH, Leow MQH, et al. Application of cabbage leaves compared to gel packs for mothers with breast engorgement: randomised controlled trial. *Int J Nurs Stud*. 2017;76:92–99

Breast Pain, Chronic >1 Week

1. Berens P, Eglash A, Malloy M, Steube AM. ABM clinical protocol #26: persistent pain with breastfeeding. *Breastfeed Med*. 2016;11(2):46–53
2. Witt AM, Burgess K, Hawn TR, Zyzanski S. Role of oral antibiotics in treatment of breastfeeding women with chronic breast pain who fail conservative therapy. *Breastfeed Med*. 2014;9(2):63–72
3. Witt AM, Mason MJ, Burgess K, Flocke S, Zyzanski S. A case control study of bacterial species and colony count in milk of breastfeeding women with chronic pain. *Breastfeed Med*. 2014;9(1):29–34

Child Care and Breastfeeding (Advice Only)

1. Witt AM, Burgess K, Hawn TR, Zyzanski S. Role of oral antibiotics in treatment of breastfeeding women with chronic breast pain who fail conservative therapy. *Breastfeed Med*. 2014;9(2):63–72
2. Colorado Department of Public Health and Environment. Breastfeeding in child care toolkit. Pueblo County, Colorado, Web site. http://county.pueblo.org/sites/default/files/documents/Breast%20Feeding%20in%20Child%20Care%20Toolkit%28Centers%29_1.pdf. Accessed April 2018

Clicking or Noisy Nursing

1. Lawrence RA, Lawrence RM. *Breastfeeding: A Guide for the Medical Profession.* 8th ed. Philadelphia, PA: Elsevier; 2016
2. Neifert M. *Great Expectations: The Essential Guide to Breastfeeding.* New York, NY: Sterling Publishing; 2009

Color Change of Human Milk

1. Anderson PO. Unusual milk colors. *Breastfeed Med.* 2018;13(3): 172–173
2. Cizmeci MN, Kanburoglu MK, Akelma AZ, Tatli MM. Rusty-pipe syndrome: a rare cause of change in the color of breastmilk. *Breastfeed Med.* 2013;8(3):340–341
3. Lawrence RA, Lawrence RM. *Breastfeeding: A Guide for the Medical Profession.* 8th ed. Philadelphia, PA: Elsevier; 2016
4. Neifert M. *Great Expectations: The Essential Guide to Breastfeeding.* New York, NY: Sterling Publishing; 2009
5. Silva JR, Carvalho R, Maia C, Osório M, Barbosa M. Rusty pipe syndrome, a cause of bloody nipple discharge: case report. *Breastfeed Med.* 2014;9(8):411–412

Constipation in the Breastfed Baby

1. Lawrence RA, Lawrence RM. *Breastfeeding: A Guide for the Medical Profession.* 8th ed. Philadelphia, PA: Elsevier; 2016
2. Schmitt BD. *Pediatric Telephone Protocols: Office Version.* 16th ed. Itasca, IL: American Academy of Pediatrics; 2019

Contraception, Lactation Amenorrhea Method (Advice Only)

1. American Academy of Pediatrics. *New Mother's Guide to Breastfeeding.* Meek JY, ed. 3rd ed. New York, NY: Bantam Books; 2017
2. Berens P, Labbok M; Academy of Breastfeeding Medicine. ABM clinical protocol #13: contraception during breastfeeding, revised 2015. *Breastfeed Med.* 2015;10:3–12
3. Hale TW, Berens P. *Clinical Therapy in Breastfeeding Patients.* 3rd ed. Amarillo, TX: Hale; 2011
4. Lawrence RA, Lawrence RM. *Breastfeeding: A Guide for the Medical Profession.* 8th ed. Philadelphia, PA: Elsevier; 2016

Cosleeping/Bed Sharing and Breastfeeding (Advice Only)

1. American Academy of Pediatrics. *New Mother's Guide to Breastfeeding.* Meek JY, ed. 3rd ed. New York, NY: Bantam Books; 2017
2. American Academy of Pediatrics Task Force on Sudden Infant Death Syndrome. SIDS and other sleep-related infant deaths: updated 2016 recommendations for a safe infant sleeping environment. *Pediatrics.* 2016;138(5):e20162938
3. Moon RY; American Academy of Pediatrics Task Force on Sudden Infant Death Syndrome. SIDS and other sleep-related infant deaths: expansion of recommendations for a safe infant sleeping environment. *Pediatrics.* 2011;128(5):1030–1039
4. Blair PS, Ball HL. The prevalence and characteristics associated with parent-infant bed-sharing in England. *Arch Dis Child.* 2004;89(12):1106–1110
5. Lawrence RA, Lawrence RM. *Breastfeeding: A Guide for the Medical Profession.* 8th ed. Philadelphia, PA: Elsevier; 2016
6. McCoy RC, Hunt CE, Lesko SM, et al. Frequency of bed sharing and its relationship to breastfeeding. *J Dev Behav Pediatr.* 2004;25(3):141–149

Distraction, Onset at 4 Months

1. Lawrence RA, Lawrence RM. *Breastfeeding: A Guide for the Medical Profession.* 8th ed. Philadelphia, PA: Elsevier; 2016
2. Neifert M. *Great Expectations: The Essential Guide to Breastfeeding.* New York, NY: Sterling Publishing; 2009

Early Weight Loss, Birth Hospital or First Week

1. Flaherman VJ, Schaefer EW, Kuzniewicz MW, Li SX, Walsh EM, Paul IM. Early weight loss nomograms for exclusively breastfed newborns. *Pediatrics.* 2015;135(1):e16–e23
2. Thulier D. Weighing the facts: a systematic review of expected patterns of weight loss in full-term, breastfed infants. *J Hum Lact.* 2016;32(1):28–34

Emotional Symptoms With Letdown

1. Cox S. A case of dysphoric milk ejection reflex (D-MER). *Breastfeed Rev.* 2010;18(1):16–18
2. D-MER.org. https://d-mer.org. Accessed March 29, 2018
3. Heise AM, Wiessinger D. Dysphoric milk ejection reflex: a case report. *Int Breastfeed J.* 2011;6(1):6

Engorgement

1. Berens P; Academy of Breastfeeding Medicine Protocol Committee. ABM clinical protocol #20: engorgement. *Breastfeed Med.* 2009;4(2):111–113
2. American Academy of Pediatrics. *New Mother's Guide to Breastfeeding.* Meek JY, ed. 3rd ed. New York, NY: Bantam Books; 2017
3. Amir LH. Managing common breastfeeding problems in the community. *BMJ.* 2014;348:g2954
4. Bolman M, Saju L, Oganesyan K, Kondrashova T, Witt AM. Recapturing the art of therapeutic breast massage during breastfeeding. *J Hum Lact.* 2013;29(3):328–331
5. Lawrence RA, Lawrence RM. *Breastfeeding: A Guide for the Medical Profession.* 8th ed. Philadelphia, PA: Elsevier; 2016
6. Mangesi L, Dowswell T. Treatments for breast engorgement during lactation. *Cochrane Database Syst Rev.* 2010;(9):CD006946
7. Neifert M. *Great Expectations: The Essential Guide to Breastfeeding.* New York, NY: Sterling Publishing; 2009

Environmental Exposures and Toxins

1. Landrigan PJ, Sonawane B, Mattison D, McCally M, Garg A. Chemical contaminants in breast milk and their impacts on children's health: an overview. *Environ Health Perspect.* 2002;110(6):A313–A315
2. Lawrence RA, Lawrence RM. *Breastfeeding: A Guide for the Medical Profession.* 8th ed. Philadelphia, PA: Elsevier; 2016
3. National Resources Defense Council. https://www.nrdc.org. Accessed March 29, 2018
4. Steingraber S. *Having Faith: An Ecologist's Journey to Motherhood.* Cambridge, MA: Perseus Publishing; 2001
5. Texas Tech University Health Sciences Center. InfantRisk Center. http://www.infantrisk.com. Accessed March 29, 2018

Exclusive Pumping

1. Casemore S. *Exclusively Pumping Breast Milk: A Guide to Providing Expressed Breast Milk for Your Baby.* 2nd ed. Napanee, Ontario: Gray Lion Publishing; 2014
2. Shealy KR, Scanlon KS, Labiner-Wolfe J, Fein SB, Grummer-Strawn LM. Characteristics of breastfeeding practices among US mothers. *Pediatrics.* 2008;122(Suppl 2):S50–S55

Expression of Human Milk: Pumping, Parts and Cleaning Equipment, Hand Expression (Advice Only)

1. American Academy of Pediatrics. *New Mother's Guide to Breastfeeding.* Meek JY, ed. 3rd ed. New York, NY: Bantam Books; 2017
2. American Academy of Pediatrics, American College of Obstetricians and Gynecologists. *Breastfeeding Handbook for Physicians.* Schanler RJ, Krebs NF, Mass SB, eds. 2nd ed. Elk Grove Village, IL: American Academy of Pediatrics; 2014

3. Consumer Reports. Breast pump buying guide. http://www. consumerreports.org/cro/breast-pumps/buying-guide.htm. Published May 2016. Accessed March 29, 2018
4. Morton J. Hand expression of breastmilk [video]. Stanford School of Medicine Web site. https://med.stanford.edu/newborns/professional-education/breastfeeding/hand-expressing-milk.html. Accessed March 29, 2018
5. US Department of Human and Health Services. Breast pumps and insurance coverage: what you need to know. HHS.gov/HealthCare Web site. https://www.womenshealth.gov/blog/breast-pumps-insurance. Accessed March 29, 2018

Fathers (Advice Only)
1. American Academy of Pediatrics. *New Mother's Guide to Breastfeeding*. Meek JY, ed. 3rd ed. New York, NY: Bantam Books; 2017
2. Goyal K, Purbiya P, Lal SN, Kaur J, Anthwal P, Puliyel JM. Correlation of infant gender with postpartum maternal and paternal depression and exclusive breastfeeding rates. *Breastfeed Med*. 2017;12:279–282
3. Kamalifard M, Hasanpoor S, Babapour Kheiroddin J, Panahi S, Bayati Payan S. Relationship between fathers' depression and perceived social support and stress in postpartum period. *J Caring Sci*. 2014;3(1):57–66
4. Neifert M. *Great Expectations: The Essential Guide to Breastfeeding*. New York, NY: Sterling Publishing; 2009
5. Pisacane A, Continisio GI, Aldinucci M, D'Amora S, Continisio P. A controlled trial of the father's role in breastfeeding promotion. *Pediatrics*. 2005;116(4):e494–e498
6. Rempel LA, Rempel JK. The breastfeeding team: the role of involved fathers in the breastfeeding family. *J Hum Lact*. 2011;27(2):115–121
7. Susin LR, Giugliani ER. Inclusion of fathers in an intervention to promote breastfeeding: impact on breastfeeding rates. *J Hum Lact*. 2008;24(4):386–392

Feeding More Frequently
1. American Academy of Pediatrics. *New Mother's Guide to Breastfeeding*. Meek JY, ed. 3rd ed. New York, NY: Bantam Books; 2017
2. Lawrence RA, Lawrence RM. *Breastfeeding: A Guide for the Medical Profession*. 8th ed. Philadelphia, PA: Elsevier; 2016
3. Neifert M. *Great Expectations: The Essential Guide to Breastfeeding*. New York, NY: Sterling Publishing; 2009

Feeding the Baby With Cleft Lip or Palate
1. American Academy of Pediatrics. *New Mother's Guide to Breastfeeding*. Meek JY, ed. 3rd ed. New York, NY: Bantam Books; 2017
2. Bessell A, Hooper L, Shaw WC, Reilly S, Reid J, Glenny AM. Feeding interventions for growth and development in infants with cleft lip, cleft palate or cleft lip and palate. *Cochrane Database Syst Rev*. 2011;(2):CD003315
3. Burianova I, Kulihova K, Vitkova V, Janota J. Breastfeeding after early repair of cleft lip in newborns with cleft lip or cleft lip and palate in a Baby-Friendly designated hospital. *J Hum Lact*. 2017;33(3):504–508
4. Lawrence RA, Lawrence RM. *Breastfeeding: A Guide for the Medical Profession*. 8th ed. Philadelphia, PA: Elsevier; 2016
5. Reilly S, Reid J, Skeat J; Academy of Breastfeeding Medicine Clinical Protocol Committee. ABM clinical protocol #17: guidelines for breastfeeding infants with cleft lip, cleft palate, or cleft lip and palate. *Breastfeed Med*. 2007;2(4):243–250

Feeding the Baby With Hypotonia
1. Lawrence RA, Lawrence RM. *Breastfeeding: A Guide for the Medical Profession*. 8th ed. Philadelphia, PA: Elsevier; 2016
2. Thomas J, Marinelli KA, Hennessy M; Academy of Breastfeeding Medicine Protocol Committee. ABM clinical protocol #16: breastfeeding the hypotonic infant. *Breastfeed Med*. 2007;2(2):112–118

Feeding the Baby With Trisomy 21 Syndrome (Down Syndrome)
1. Centers for Disease Control and Prevention. Learn about *Cronobacter* infection. http://www.cdc.gov/Features/Cronobacter. Updated April 10, 2017. Accessed March 29, 2018
2. Lawrence RA, Lawrence RM. *Breastfeeding: A Guide for the Medical Profession*. 8th ed. Philadelphia, PA: Elsevier; 2016
3. Pisacane A, Toscano E, Pirri I, et al. Down syndrome and breastfeeding. *Acta Paediatr*. 2003;92(12):1479–1481
4. Thomas J, Marinelli KA, Hennessy M; Academy of Breastfeeding Medicine Protocol Committee. ABM clinical protocol #16: breastfeeding the hypotonic infant. *Breastfeed Med*. 2007;2(2):112–118

Fortification of Human Milk Recipes (Advice Only)
1. Centers for Disease Control and Prevention. Learn about *Cronobacter* infection. http://www.cdc.gov/Features/Cronobacter. Updated April 10, 2017. Accessed March 29, 2018
2. Groh-Wargo S, Sapsford A. Enteral nutrition support of the preterm infant in the neonatal intensive care unit. *Nutr Clin Pract*. 2009;24(3):363–376
3. Lainwala S, Kosyakova N, Spizzoucco AM, Herson V, Brownell EA. Clinical and nutritional outcomes of two liquid human milk fortifiers for premature infants. *J Neonatal Perinatal Med*. 2017;10(4):393–401
4. McCormick FM, Henderson G, Fahey T, McGuire W. Multinutrient fortification of human breast milk for preterm infants following hospital discharge. *Cochrane Database Syst Rev*. 2010;(7):CD004866
5. Ziegler EE. Human milk and human milk fortifiers. *World Rev Nutr Diet*. 2014;110:215–227

Fussiness, Colic, and Crying in the Breastfed Baby
1. Caffeine Informer. Caffeine content of drinks. http://www.caffeineinformer.com/the-caffeine-database. Accessed March 29, 2018
2. Erikson Institute. Fussy Baby Network Web site. https://www.erikson.edu/fussy-baby-network. Accessed March 29, 2018
3. Evans RW, Fergusson DM, Allardyce RA, Taylor B. Maternal diet and infantile colic in breast-fed infants. *Lancet*. 1981;1(8234):1340–1342
4. Garrison MM, Christakis DA. A systematic review of treatments for infant colic. *Pediatrics*. 2000;106(1 Pt 2):184–190
5. Karp H. *The Happiest Baby on the Block: The New Way to Calm Crying and Help Your Newborn Baby Sleep Longer*. 2nd ed. New York, NY: Bantam Books; 2015
6. Pease AS, Fleming PJ, Hauck FR, et al. Swaddling and the risk of sudden infant death syndrome: a meta-analysis. *Pediatrics*. 2016;137(6):e20153275
7. Schmitt BD. *Pediatric Telephone Protocols: Office Version*. 16th ed. Itasca, IL: American Academy of Pediatrics; 2019
8. School of Babywearing. The T.I.C.K.S. rule for safe babywearing. http://www.schoolofbabywearing.com/Images/TICKS.pdf. Accessed March 29, 2018

Gassiness in the Breastfed Baby
1. Evans RW, Fergusson DM, Allardyce RA, Taylor B. Maternal diet and infantile colic in breast-fed infants. *Lancet*. 1981;1(8234):1340–1342
2. Lawrence RA, Lawrence RM. *Breastfeeding: A Guide for the Medical Profession*. 8th ed. Philadelphia, PA: Elsevier; 2016

3. Mayo Clinic Staff. Breast rash. Causes Mayo Clinic Web site. https://www.mayoclinic.org/symptoms/breast-rash/basics/causes/sym-20050817. Published January 11, 2018. Accessed March 29, 2018

4. Neifert M. *Great Expectations: The Essential Guide to Breastfeeding.* New York, NY: Sterling Publishing; 2009

Jaundice, Newborn

1. Azzuqa A, Watchko JF. Scleral (conjunctival) icterus in neonates: a marker of significant hyperbilirubinemia. *E-PAS.* 2013:3841.708

2. Bhutani VK, Johnson LM, Keren R. Treating acute bilirubin encephalopathy—before it's too late. *Contemp Pediatr.* 2005;22(5):57–74

3. Brumbaugh D, Mack C. Conjugated hyperbilirubinemia in children. *Pediatr Rev.* 2012;33(7):291–302

4. Kuzniewicz MW, Wickremasinghe AC, Wu YW, et al. Incidence, etiology, and outcomes of hazardous hyperbilirubinemia in newborns. *Pediatrics.* 2014;134(3):504–509

5. Maisels MJ. Transcutaneous bilirubin measurement: does it work in the real world? *Pediatrics.* 2015;135(2):364–366

6. Maisels MJ, Clune S, Coleman K, et al. The natural history of jaundice in predominantly breastfed infants. *Pediatrics.* 2014;134(2):e340–e345

7. US Preventive Services Task Force. Screening of infants for hyperbilirubinemia to prevent chronic bilirubin encephalopathy: US Preventive Services Task Force recommendation statement. *Pediatrics.* 2009;124(4):1172–1177

Late Preterm Newborn

1. Academy of Breastfeeding Medicine. ABM clinical protocol #10: breastfeeding the late preterm infant (34(0/7) to 36(6/7) weeks gestation) (first revision June 2011). *Breastfeed Med.* 2011;6(3):151–156

2. American Academy of Pediatrics. *New Mother's Guide to Breastfeeding.* Meek JY, ed. 3rd ed. New York, NY: Bantam Books; 2017

3. Lawrence RA, Lawrence RM. *Breastfeeding: A Guide for the Medical Profession.* 8th ed. Philadelphia, PA: Elsevier; 2016

4. McKechnie AC, Eglash A. Nipple shields: a review of the literature. *Breastfeed Med.* 2010;5(6):309–314

5. Walker M. Breastfeeding the late preterm infant. *J Obstet Gynecol Neonatal Nurs.* 2008;37(6):692–701

6. Wright NE. Breastfeeding the borderline (near term) preterm infant. *Breastfeed Rev.* 2004;12(3):17–24

Lifestyle or Personal Care Questions (Advice Only)

1. Buser GL, Mató S, Zhang AY, Metcalf BJ, Beall B, Thomas AR. Notes from the field: late-onset infant group B streptococcus infection associated with maternal consumption of capsules containing dehydrated placenta - Oregon, 2016. *MMWR Morb Mortal Wkly Rep.* 2017;66(25):677–678

2. Caffeine Informer. Caffeine content of drinks. http://www.caffeineinformer.com/the-caffeine-database. Accessed March 29, 2018

3. Centers for Disease Control and Prevention. Breastfeeding. Travel recommendations for the nursing mother. http://www.cdc.gov/breastfeeding/recommendations/travel_recommendations.htm. Updated June 17, 2015. Accessed March 29, 2018

4. Garbin CP, Deacon JP, Rowan MK, Hartmann PE, Geddes DT. Association of nipple piercing with abnormal milk production and breastfeeding. *JAMA.* 2009;301(24):2550–2551

5. Hale TW, Berens P. *Clinical Therapy in Breastfeeding Patients.* 3rd ed. Amarillo, TX: Hale; 2011

6. Harrison D, Reszel J, Bueno M, et al. Breastfeeding for procedural pain in infants beyond the neonatal period. *Cochrane Database Syst Rev.* 2016;(10):CD011248

7. Lawrence RA, Lawrence RM. *Breastfeeding: A Guide for the Medical Profession.* 8th ed. Philadelphia, PA: Elsevier; 2016

8. Martin J. Is nipple piercing compatible with breastfeeding? *J Hum Lact.* 2004;20(3):319–321

9. Millner VS, Eichold BH 2nd. Body piercing and tattooing perspectives. *Clin Nurse Res.* 2001;10(4):424–441

10. Mohrbacher N, Stock J. *The Breastfeeding Answer Book.* 3rd rev ed. Schaumburg, IL: La Leche League International; 2003

11. Şener Taplak A, Erdem E. A comparison of breast milk and sucrose in reducing neonatal pain during eye exam for retinopathy of prematurity. *Breastfeed Med.* 2017;12:305–310

12. Shah PS, Herbozo C, Aliwalas LL, Shah VS. Breastfeeding or breast milk for procedural pain in neonates. *Cochrane Database Syst Rev.* 2012;(12):CD004950

13. Texas Tech University Health Sciences Center. InfantRisk Center. http://www.infantrisk.com. Accessed March 29, 2018

14. Transportation Security Administration, US Department of Homeland Security. Traveling with children. https://www.tsa.gov/travel/special-procedures/traveling-children. Accessed March 29, 2018

Long-term Breastfeeding (Advice Only)

1. American Academy of Pediatrics Section on Breastfeeding. Breastfeeding and the use of human milk. *Pediatrics.* 2012;129(3):e827–e841

2. Lawrence RA, Lawrence RM. *Breastfeeding: A Guide for the Medical Profession.* 8th ed. Philadelphia, PA: Elsevier; 2016

3. Neifert M. *Great Expectations: The Essential Guide to Breastfeeding.* New York, NY: Sterling Publishing; 2009

4. World Health Organization. Health topics: breastfeeding. http://www.who.int/topics/breastfeeding/en. Accessed March 29, 2018

Low Milk Supply

1. Academy of Breastfeeding Medicine Protocol Committee. ABM clinical protocol #3: hospital guidelines for the use of supplementary feedings in the healthy term breastfed neonate, revised 2009. *Breastfeed Med.* 2009;4(3):175–182

2. Academy of Breastfeeding Medicine Protocol Committee. ABM clinical protocol #9: use of galactogogues in initiating or augmenting the rate of maternal milk secretion (first revision January 2011). *Breastfeed Med.* 2011;6(1):41–49

3. Asztalos EV, Campbell-Yeo M, da Silva OP, et al. Enhancing human milk production with domperidone in mothers of preterm infants. *J Hum Lact.* 2017;33(1):181–187

4. Bunik M, Shobe P, O'Connor ME, et al. Are 2 weeks of daily breastfeeding support insufficient to overcome the influences of formula? *Acad Pediatr.* 2010;10(1):21–28

5. Buntuchai G, Pavadhgul P, Kittipichai W, Satheannoppakao W. Traditional galactagogue foods and their connection to human milk volume in Thai breastfeeding mothers. *J Hum Lact.* 2017;33(3):552–559

6. Flaherman VJ, Schaefer EW, Kuzniewicz MW, Li SX, Walsh EM, Paul IM. Early weight loss nomograms for exclusively breastfed newborns. *Pediatrics.* 2015;135(1):e16–e23

7. Gatti L. Maternal perceptions of insufficient milk supply in breastfeeding. *J Nurs Scholarsh.* 2008;40(4):355–363

8. Lawrence RA, Lawrence RM. *Breastfeeding: A Guide for the Medical Profession.* 8th ed. Philadelphia, PA: Elsevier; 2016

9. Neifert M. *Great Expectations: The Essential Guide to Breastfeeding.* New York, NY: Sterling Publishing; 2009

10. Paul C, Zénut M, Dorut A, et al. Use of domperidone as a galactagogue drug: a systematic review of the benefit-risk ratio. *J Hum Lact.* 2015;31(1):57–63
11. Sacco LM, Caulfield LE, Gittelsohn J, Martínez H. The conceptualization of perceived insufficient milk among Mexican mothers. *J Hum Lact.* 2006;22(3):277–286
12. Thulier D. Weighing the facts: a systematic review of expected patterns of weight loss in full-term, breastfed infants. *J Hum Lact.* 2016;32(1):28–34

Marijuana Use

1. Hale TW, Rowe HE. *Medications and Mothers' Milk 2017.* New York, NY: Springer Publishing Co; 2017
2. Jaques SC, Kingsbury A, Henshcke P, et al. Cannabis, the pregnant woman and her child: weeding out the myths. *J Perinatol.* 2014;34(6):417–424
3. Klonoff-Cohen H, Lam-Kruglick P. Maternal and paternal recreational drug use and sudden infant death syndrome. *Arch Pediatr Adolesc Med.* 2001;155(7):765–770

Maternal Anesthesia/Analgesia (Advice Only)

1. Anderson PO. Choosing medication alternatives during breastfeeding, avoiding alternative facts. *Breastfeed Med.* 2017;12(6):328–330
2. Hale TW, Berens P. *Clinical Therapy in Breastfeeding Patients.* 3rd ed. Amarillo, TX: Hale; 2011
3. Lawrence RA, Lawrence RM. *Breastfeeding: A Guide for the Medical Profession.* 8th ed. Philadelphia, PA: Elsevier; 2016
4. Montgomery A, Hale TW; Academy of Breastfeeding Medicine Protocol Committee. ABM clinical protocol #15: analgesia and anesthesia for the breastfeeding mother. *Breastfeed Med.* 2006;1(4):271–277
5. Texas Tech University Health Sciences Center. InfantRisk Center. http://www.infantrisk.com. Accessed March 29, 2018
6. US Food and Drug Administration. FDA drug safety communication: FDA requires labeling changes for prescription opioid cough and cold medicines to limit their use to adults 18 years and older. https://www.fda.gov/Safety/MedWatch/SafetyInformation/SafetyAlertsforHumanMedicalProducts/ucm592053.htm. Accessed March 29, 2018

Maternal Contraindications/Causes for Concern With Breastfeeding (Advice Only)

1. American Academy of Pediatrics. *Red Book: 2018–2021 Report of the Committee on Infectious Diseases.* Kimberlin DW, Brady MT, Jackson MA, Long SS, eds. 31st ed. Itasca, IL: American Academy of Pediatrics; 2018
2. Bausch DG, Towner JS, Dowell SF, et al. Assessment of the risk of Ebola virus transmission from bodily fluids and fomites. *J Infect Dis.* 2007;196(Suppl 2):S142–S147
3. Centers for Disease Control and Prevention. Ebola: Ebola virus disease; recommendations for breastfeeding/infant feeding in the context of Ebola virus disease. https://www.cdc.gov/vhf/ebola/hcp/recommendations-breastfeeding-infant-feeding-ebola.html. Updated June 10, 2016. Accessed March 29, 2018
4. Colt S, Garcia-Casal MN, Peña-Rosas JP, et al. Transmission of Zika virus through breast milk and other breastfeeding-related bodily-fluids: a systematic review. *PLoS Negl Trop Dis.* 2017;11(4):e0005528
5. Ebola haemorrhagic fever in Zaire, 1976. *Bull World Health Organ.* 1978;56(2):271–293
6. Hale TW, Berens P. *Clinical Therapy in Breastfeeding Patients.* 3rd ed. Amarillo, TX: Hale; 2011

7. Hale TW, Rowe HE. *Medications and Mothers' Milk 2017.* New York, NY: Springer Publishing Co; 2017
8. Lawrence RA, Lawrence RM. *Breastfeeding: A Guide for the Medical Profession.* 8th ed. Philadelphia, PA: Elsevier; 2016
9. Neifert M. *Great Expectations: The Essential Guide to Breastfeeding.* New York, NY: Sterling Publishing; 2009
10. Texas Tech University Health Sciences Center. InfantRisk Center. http://www.infantrisk.com. Accessed March 29, 2018
11. US National Library of Medicine. Toxnet Toxicology Database Network. http://www.toxnet.nlm.nih.gov. Accessed March 29, 2018
12. WHO Collaborative Study Team on the Role of Breastfeeding on the Prevention of Infant Mortality. Effect of breastfeeding on infant and child mortality due to infectious diseases in less developed counties: a pooled analysis. *Lancet.* 2000;355(9202):451–455

Maternal Illnesses (Advice Only)

1. American Academy of Pediatrics. *Red Book: 2018–2021 Report of the Committee on Infectious Diseases.* Kimberlin DW, Brady MT, Jackson MA, Long SS, eds. 31st ed. Itasca, IL: American Academy of Pediatrics; 2018
2. Centers for Disease Control and Prevention. Breastfeeding. Vaccinations. http://www.cdc.gov/breastfeeding/recommendations/vaccinations.htm. Updated August 25, 2015. Accessed March 29, 2018
3. Drayton BA, Patterson JA, Nippita TA, Ford JB. Red blood cell transfusion after postpartum haemorrhage and breastmilk feeding at discharge: a population-based study. *Aust N Z J Obstet Gynaecol.* 2016;56(6):591–598
4. Hale TW, Berens P. *Clinical Therapy in Breastfeeding Patients.* 3rd ed. Amarillo, TX: Hale; 2011
5. Lawrence RA, Lawrence RM. *Breastfeeding: A Guide for the Medical Profession.* 8th ed. Philadelphia, PA: Elsevier; 2016
6. Marraccini ME, Weyandt LL, Gudmundsdottir BG, Oster DR, McCallum A. Attention-deficit hyperactivity disorder: clinical considerations for women. *J Midwifery Womens Health.* 2017;62(6):684–695
7. Meador KJ, Baker GA, Browning N, et al. Breastfeeding in children of women taking antiepileptic drugs: cognitive outcomes at age 6 years. *JAMA Pediatr.* 2014;168(8):729–736
8. Texas Tech University Health Sciences Center. InfantRisk Center. http://www.infantrisk.com. Accessed March 29, 2018

Maternal Ingestion of Foods and Herbs (Advice Only)

1. Academy of Breastfeeding Medicine Protocol Committee. ABM clinical protocol #9: use of galactogogues in initiating or augmenting the rate of maternal milk secretion (first revision January 2011). *Breastfeed Med.* 2011;6(1):41–49
2. Berti C, Agostoni C, Davanzo R, et al. Early-life nutritional exposures and lifelong health: immediate and long-lasting impacts of probiotics, vitamin D, and breastfeeding. *Nutr Rev.* 2017;75(2):83–97
3. Hurtado JA, Maldonado-Lobón JA, Díaz-Ropero MP, et al. Oral administration to nursing women of *Lactobacillus fermentum* CECT5716 prevents lactational mastitis development: a randomized controlled trial. *Breastfeed Med.* 2017;12(4):202–209
4. Institute for Agriculture and Trade Policy. Food and health. https://www.iatp.org/issue/health/food/food-and-health. Accessed March 29, 2018
5. Lawrence RA, Lawrence RM. *Breastfeed: A Guide for the Medical Profession.* 8th ed. Philadelphia, PA: Elsevier; 2016
6. Neifert M. *Great Expectations: The Essential Guide to Breastfeeding.* New York, NY: Sterling Publishing; 2009

7. US Food and Drug Administration. GRAS notice inventory. https://www.fda.gov/Food/IngredientsPackagingLabeling/GRAS/NoticeInventory/default.htm. Accessed March 29, 2018

Maternal Medications (Advice Only)

1. Datta P, Rewers-Felkins K, Kallem RR, Baker T, Hale TW. Transfer of low dose aspirin into human milk. *J Hum Lact.* 2017;33(2):296–299
2. Hale TW, Berens P. *Clinical Therapy in Breastfeeding Patients.* 3rd ed. Amarillo, TX: Hale; 2011
3. Hale TW, Rowe HE. *Medications and Mothers' Milk 2017.* New York, NY: Springer Publishing Co; 2017
4. Lawrence RA, Lawrence RM. *Breastfeeding: A Guide for the Medical Profession.* 8th ed. Philadelphia, PA: Elsevier; 2016
5. Neifert M. *Great Expectations: The Essential Guide to Breastfeeding.* New York, NY: Sterling Publishing; 2009
6. Texas Tech University Health Sciences Center. InfantRisk Center. http://www.infantrisk.com. Accessed March 29, 2018
7. US National Library of Medicine. Toxnet Toxicology Data Network Drugs and Lactation Database (LactMed). http://toxnet.nlm.nih.gov/newtoxnet/lactmed.htm. Accessed March 29, 2018

Maternal Methicillin-Resistant *Staphylococcal aureus*

1. Amir LH; Academy of Breastfeeding Medicine Protocol Committee. ABM clinical protocol #4: mastitis, revised March 2014. *Breastfeed Med.* 2014;9(5):239–243
2. Sheybani F, Sarvghad M, Naderi H, Gharib M. Treatment for and clinical characteristics of granulomatous mastitis. *Obstet Gynecol.* 2015;125(4):801–807
3. US National Library of Medicine. Toxnet Toxicology Data Network Drugs and Lactation Database (LactMed). http://toxnet.nlm.nih.gov/newtoxnet/lactmed.htm. Accessed March 29, 2018

Maternal Postpartum Depression

1. Academy of Breastfeeding Medicine Protocol Committee. ABM clinical protocol #18: use of antidepressants in nursing mothers. *Breastfeed Med.* 2008;3(1):44–52
2. Cox JL, Holden JM, Sagovsky R. Detection of postnatal depression. Development of the 10-item Edinburgh Postnatal Depression Scale. *Br J Psychiatry.* 1987;150:782–786
3. Hale TW, Berens P. *Clinical Therapy in Breastfeeding Patients.* 3rd ed. Amarillo, TX: Hale; 2011
4. Kendall-Tackett K, Hale TW. The use of antidepressants in pregnant and breastfeeding women: a review of recent studies. *J Hum Lact.* 2010;26(2):187–195
5. Lawrence RA, Lawrence RM. *Breastfeeding: A Guide for the Medical Profession.* 8th ed. Philadelphia, PA: Elsevier; 2016

Maternal Postpartum Vaginal Bleeding

1. Lawrence RA, Lawrence RM. *Breastfeeding: A Guide for the Medical Profession.* 8th ed. Philadelphia, PA: Elsevier; 2016
2. Long VE, McMullen PC. *Telephone Triage for Obstetrics & Gynecology.* 2nd ed. Philadelphia, PA: Lippincott Williams & Wilkins; 2010
3. Oyelese Y, Ananth CV. Postpartum hemorrhage: epidemiology, risk factors, and causes. *Clin Obstet Gynecol.* 2010;53(1):147–156

Maternal Smoking, Vaping, and Cessation Strategies

1. Almas S. E-cigarettes: a review on composition, safety, and efficacy as smoking cessation aids. InfantRisk Center Web site. https://www.infantrisk.com/content/e-cigarettes-review-composition-safety-and-efficacy-smoking-cessation-aids. Accessed March 29, 2018
2. American Academy of Pediatrics. *New Mother's Guide to Breastfeeding.* Meek JY, ed. 3rd ed. New York, NY: Bantam Books; 2017

3. Lawrence RA, Lawrence RM. *Breastfeeding: A Guide for the Medical Profession.* 8th ed. Philadelphia, PA: Elsevier; 2016

Milk Leaking From Newborn's Breasts (Galactorrhea)

Madlon-Kay DJ. 'Witch's milk'. Galactorrhea in the newborn. *Am J Dis Child.* 1986;140(3):252–253

Milk Storage and Return to Work/School

1. Eglash A; Academy of Breastfeeding Medicine Protocol Committee. ABM clinical protocol #8: human milk storage information for home use for full-term infants (original protocol March 2004; revision #1 March 2010). *Breastfeed Med.* 2010;5(3):127–130
2. American Academy of Pediatrics. *New Mother's Guide to Breastfeeding.* Meek JY, ed. 3rd ed. New York, NY: Bantam Books; 2017
3. Centers for Disease Control and Prevention. Proper handling and storage of human milk. https://www.cdc.gov/breastfeeding/recommendations/handling_breastmilk.htm. Updated March 21, 2018. Accessed March 29, 2018
4. Colburn-Smith C, Serrette A. *The Milk Memos: How Real Moms Learned to Mix Business with Babies—and How You Can, Too.* New York, NY: Penguin Group; 2007
5. Colorado Breastfeeding Coalition. http://www.cobfc.org. Accessed March 29, 2018
6. Eglash A, Simon L; Academy of Breastfeeding Medicine. ABM clinical protocol #8: human milk storage information for home use for full-term infants, revised 2017. *Breastfeed Med.* 2017;12(7):390–395
7. Lawrence RA, Lawrence RM. *Breastfeeding: A Guide for the Medical Profession.* 8th ed. Philadelphia, PA: Elsevier; 2016
8. Neifert M. *Great Expectations: The Essential Guide to Breastfeeding.* New York, NY: Sterling Publishing; 2009
9. US Breastfeeding Committee. Workplace support in federal law. http://www.usbreastfeeding.org/workplace-law. Accessed March 29, 2018

Mistaken Milk Ingestion, Milk Sharing

1. Centers for Disease Control and Prevention. Breastfeeding. What to do if an infant or child is mistakenly fed another woman's expressed breast milk. http://www.cdc.gov/breastfeeding/recommendations/other_mothers_milk.htm. Updated May 31, 2016. Accessed March 29, 2018
2. Kair LR, Colaizy TT, Hubbard D, Flaherman VJ. Donor milk in the newborn nursery at the University of Iowa Children's Hospital. *Breastfeed Med.* 2014;9(10):547–550
3. Kair LR, Flaherman VJ. Donor milk or formula: a qualitative study of postpartum mothers of healthy newborns. *J Hum Lact.* 2017; 33(4):710–716
4. Keim SA, Hogan JS, McNamara KA, et al. Microbial contamination of human milk purchased via the Internet. *Pediatrics.* 2013; 132(5):e1227–e1235
5. Keim SA, McNamara KA, Dillon CE, et al. Breastmilk sharing: awareness and participation among women in the Moms2Moms Study. *Breastfeed Med.* 2014;9(8):398–406
6. Keim SA, McNamara KA, Jayadeva CM, Braun AC, Dillon CE, Geraghty SR. Breast milk sharing via the internet: the practice and health and safety considerations. *Matern Child Health J.* 2014;18(6):1471–1479

Multiples (Advice Only)

1. American Academy of Pediatrics. *New Mother's Guide to Breastfeeding.* Meek JY, ed. 3rd ed. New York, NY: Bantam Books; 2017
2. Geraghty SR, Khoury JC, Kalkwarf HJ. Comparison of feeding among multiple birth infants. *Twin Res.* 2004;7(6):542–547
3. Geraghty SR, Khoury JC, Kalkwarf HJ. Human milk pumping rates of mothers of singletons and mothers of multiples. *J Hum Lact.* 2005;21(4):413–420

4. Lawrence RA, Lawrence RM. *Breastfeeding: A Guide for the Medical Profession*. 8th ed. Philadelphia, PA: Elsevier; 2016

5. Neifert M. *Great Expectations: The Essential Guide to Breastfeeding*. New York, NY: Sterling Publishing; 2009

Newborn Contraindications to Breastfeeding (Advice Only)

1. American Academy of Pediatrics. *New Mother's Guide to Breastfeeding*. Meek JY, ed. 3rd ed. New York, NY: Bantam Books; 2017

2. Kose E, Aksoy B, Kuyum P, Tuncer N, Arslan N, Ozturk Y. The effects of breastfeeding in infants with phenylketonuria. *J Pediatr Nurs*. 2018;38:27–32

3. Lawrence RA, Lawrence RM. *Breastfeeding: A Guide for the Medical Profession*. 8th ed. Philadelphia, PA: Elsevier; 2016

Nipple Abnormality: Flat/Short, Inverted, Large, or Bulbous

1. American Academy of Pediatrics. *New Mother's Guide to Breastfeeding*. Meek JY, ed. 3rd ed. New York, NY: Bantam Books; 2017

2. Lawrence RA, Lawrence RM. *Breastfeeding: A Guide for the Medical Profession*. 8th ed. Philadelphia, PA: Elsevier; 2016

3. Neifert M. *Great Expectations: The Essential Guide to Breastfeeding*. New York, NY: Sterling Publishing; 2009

4. Walker M. Conquering common breast-feeding problems. *J Perinat Neonatal Nurs*. 2008;22(4):267–274

No Latch or Inability to Latch

1. Lawrence RA, Lawrence RM. *Breastfeeding: A Guide for the Medical Profession*. 8th ed. Philadelphia, PA: Elsevier; 2016

2. Neifert M. *Great Expectations: The Essential Guide to Breastfeeding*. New York, NY: Sterling Publishing; 2009

Nursing Strike or Refusal

1. American Academy of Pediatrics. *New Mother's Guide to Breastfeeding*. Meek JY, ed. 3rd ed. New York, NY: Bantam Books; 2017

2. Lawrence RA, Lawrence RM. *Breastfeeding: A Guide for the Medical Profession*. 8th ed. Philadelphia, PA: Elsevier; 2016

3. Neifert M. *Great Expectations: The Essential Guide to Breastfeeding*. New York, NY: Sterling Publishing; 2009

Nursing With Pregnancy

1. Flower H. *Adventures in Tandem Nursing: Breastfeeding During Pregnancy and Beyond*. Schaumburg, IL: La Leche League International; 2003

2. Lawrence RA, Lawrence RM. *Breastfeeding: A Guide for the Medical Profession*. 8th ed. Philadelphia, PA: Elsevier; 2016

3. Neifert M. *Great Expectations: The Essential Guide to Breastfeeding*. New York, NY: Sterling Publishing; 2009

Overactive Letdown/Overabundant Milk Supply

1. Lawrence RA, Lawrence RM. *Breastfeeding: A Guide for the Medical Profession*. 8th ed. Philadelphia, PA: Elsevier; 2016

2. Livingstone V. Too much of a good thing. Maternal and infant hyperlactation syndromes. *Can Fam Physician*. 1996;42:89–99

3. Neifert M. *Great Expectations: The Essential Guide to Breastfeeding*. New York, NY: Sterling Publishing; 2009

4. van Veldhuizen-Staas CG. Overabundant milk supply: an alternative way to intervene by full drainage and block feeding. *Int Breastfeed J*. 2007;2:11

Pacifiers and Slow-Flow Nipples (Advice Only)

1. Academy of Breastfeeding Medicine Protocol Committee. ABM clinical protocol #3: hospital guidelines for the use of supplementary feedings in the healthy term breastfed neonate, revised 2009. *Breastfeed Med*. 2009;4(3):175–182

2. Lawrence RA, Lawrence RM. *Breastfeeding: A Guide for the Medical Profession*. 8th ed. Philadelphia, PA: Elsevier; 2016

3. Neifert M. *Great Expectations: The Essential Guide to Breastfeeding*. New York, NY: Sterling Publishing; 2009

4. Schmitt BD. *Pediatric Telephone Protocols: Office Version*. 16th ed. Itasca, IL: American Academy of Pediatrics; 2019

5. Sipsma HL, Kornfeind K, Kair LR. Pacifiers and exclusive breastfeeding: does risk for postpartum depression modify the association? *J Hum Lact*. 2017;33(4):692–700

Referral to Local Resources (Advice Only)

1. American Academy of Pediatrics. *New Mother's Guide to Breastfeeding*. Meek JY, ed. 3rd ed. New York, NY: Bantam Books; 2017

2. Lawrence RA, Lawrence RM. *Breastfeeding: A Guide for the Medical Profession*. 8th ed. Philadelphia, PA: Elsevier; 2016

3. Neifert M. *Great Expectations: The Essential Guide to Breastfeeding*. New York, NY: Sterling Publishing; 2009

Refusing Bottle, Preferring to Nurse

1. American Academy of Pediatrics. *New Mother's Guide to Breastfeeding*. Meek JY, ed. 3rd ed. New York, NY: Bantam Books; 2017

2. Lawrence RA, Lawrence RM. *Breastfeeding: A Guide for the Medical Profession*. 8th ed. Philadelphia, PA: Elsevier; 2016

3. Neifert M. *Great Expectations: The Essential Guide to Breastfeeding*. New York, NY: Sterling Publishing; 2009

Sleepy Newborn

1. Home RS, Parslow PM, Ferens D, Watts AM, Adamson TM. Comparison of evoked arousability in breast and formula fed infants. *Arch Dis Child*. 2004;89(1):22–25

2. Home RS, Sly DJ, Cranage SM, Chau B, Adamson TM. Effects of prematurity on arousal from sleep in the newborn infant. *Pediatr Res*. 2000;47(4 Pt 1):468–474

Sore Nipples

1. Alexander A, Dowling D, Furman L. What do pregnant low-income women say about breastfeeding? *Breastfeed Med*. 2010;5(1):17–23

2. American Academy of Pediatrics. *New Mother's Guide to Breastfeeding*. Meek JY, ed. 3rd ed. New York, NY: Bantam Books; 2017

3. Heller MM, Fullerton-Stone H, Murase JE. Caring for new mothers: diagnosis, management and treatment of nipple dermatitis in breastfeeding mothers. *Int J Dermatol*. 2012;51(10):1149–1161

4. Lawrence RA, Lawrence RM. *Breastfeeding: A Guide for the Medical Profession*. 8th ed. Philadelphia, PA: Elsevier; 2016

5. Neifert M. *Great Expectations: The Essential Guide to Breastfeeding*. New York, NY: Sterling Publishing; 2009

6. Nommsen-Rivers LA, Chantry CJ, Cohen RJ, Dewey KG. Comfort with the idea of formula feeding helps explain ethnic disparity in breastfeeding intentions among expectant first-time mothers. *Breastfeed Med*. 2010;5(1):25–33

7. Walker M. Conquering common breast-feeding problems. *J Perinat Neonatal Nurs*. 2008;22(4):267–274

Spitting Up (Reflux)

1. Hassall E. Over-prescription of acid-suppressing medications in infants: how it came about, why it's wrong, and what to do about it. *J Pediatr.* 2012;160(2):193–198
2. Lightdale JR, Gremse DA; American Academy of Pediatrics Section on Gastroenterology, Hepatology, and Nutrition. Gastroesophageal reflux: management guidance for the pediatrician. *Pediatrics.* 2013;131(5):e1684–e1695
3. Rosen R. Gastroesophageal reflux in infants more than just a pHenomenon. *JAMA Pediatr.* 2014;168(1):83–89
4. Scherer LD, Zikmund-Fisher BJ, Fagerline A, Tarini BA. Influence of "GERD" label on parents' decision to medicate infants. *Pediatrics.* 2013;131(5):839–845
5. van der Pol R, Langendam M, Benninga M, van Wijk M, Tabbers M. Efficacy and safety of histamine-2 receptor antagonists. *JAMA Pediatr.* 2014;168(10):947–954

Substances of Abuse (Illicit Drugs)

1. Jansson LM; Academy of Breastfeeding Medicine Protocol Committee. ABM clinical protocol #21: guidelines for breastfeeding and the drug-dependent woman. *Breastfeed Med.* 2009;4(4):225–228
2. Hale TW, Berens P. *Clinical Therapy in Breastfeeding Patients.* 3rd ed. Amarillo, TX: Hale; 2011
3. Hale TW, Rowe HE. *Medications and Mothers' Milk 2017.* New York, NY: Springer Publishing Co; 2017
4. Lawrence RA, Lawrence RM. *Breastfeeding: A Guide for the Medical Profession.* 8th ed. Philadelphia, PA: Elsevier; 2016
5. Texas Tech University Health Sciences Center. InfantRisk Center. http://www.infantrisk.com. Accessed March 29, 2018
6. US Department of Health and Human Services. Results from the 2016 National Survey on Drug Use and Health: summary of national findings. Substance Abuse and Mental Health Service Administration Web site. https://www.samhsa.gov/samhsa-data-outcomes-quality/major-data-collections/reports-detailed-tables-2016-NSDUH. Accessed March 29, 2018
7. US National Library of Medicine. Toxnet Toxicology Data Network Drug and Lactation Database (LactMed). http://toxnet.nlm.nih.gov/newtoxnet/lactmed.htm. Accessed March 29, 2018

Tandem Nursing

1. American Academy of Pediatrics. *New Mother's Guide to Breastfeeding.* Meek JY, ed. 3rd ed. New York, NY: Bantam Books; 2017
2. Flower H. *Adventures in Tandem Nursing: Breastfeeding During Pregnancy and Beyond.* Schaumburg, IL: La Leche League International; 2003
3. Lawrence RA, Lawrence RM. *Breastfeeding: A Guide for the Medical Profession.* 8th ed. Philadelphia, PA: Elsevier; 2016

Taste Change of Human Milk

1. American Academy of Pediatrics. *New Mother's Guide to Breastfeeding.* Meek JY, ed. 3rd ed. New York, NY: Bantam Books; 2017
2. Lawrence RA, Lawrence RM. *Breastfeeding: A Guide for the Medical Profession.* 8th ed. Philadelphia, PA: Elsevier; 2016
3. Neifert M. *Great Expectations: The Essential Guide to Breastfeeding.* New York, NY: Sterling Publishing; 2009

Tongue-tie

1. Academy of Breastfeeding Medicine Protocol Committee. ABM clinical protocol #11: neonatal ankyloglossia. *Breastfeed Med.*
2. Bin-Nun A, Kasirer YM, Mimouni FB. A dramatic increase in tongue tie-related articles: a 67 years systematic review. *Breastfeed Med.* 2017;12(7):410–414

3. Buryk M, Bloom D, Shope T. Efficacy of neonatal release of ankyloglossia: a randomized trial. *Pediatrics.* 2011;128(2):280–288
4. Geddes DT, Langton DB, Gollow I, Jacobs LA, Hartmann PE, Simmer K. Frenulotomy for breastfeeding infants with ankyloglossia: effect on milk removal and sucking mechanism as imaged by ultrasound. *Pediatrics.* 2008;122(1):e188–e194
5. Haham A, Marom R, Mangel L, Botzer E, Dollberg S. Prevalence of breastfeeding difficulties in newborns with a lingual frenulum: a prospective cohort series. *Breastfeed Med.* 2014;9(9):438–441
6. Lawrence RA, Lawrence RM. *Breastfeeding: A Guide for the Medical Profession.* 8th ed. Philadelphia, PA: Elsevier; 2016
7. Messner AH, Lalakea ML, Aby J, Macmahon J, Bair E. Ankyloglossia: incidence and associated feeding difficulties. *Arch Otolaryngol Head Neck Surg.* 2000;126(1):36–39
8. O'Shea JE, Foster JP, O'Donnell CP, et al. Frenotomy for tongue-tie in newborn infants. *Cochrane Database Syst Rev.* 2017;(3):CD011065
9. Power RF, Murphy JF. Tongue-tie and frenotomy in infants with breastfeeding difficulties: achieving a balance. *Arch Dis Child.* 2015;100(5):489–494
10. Walsh J, Tunkel D. Diagnosis and treatment of ankyloglossia in newborns and infants: a review. *JAMA Otolaryngol Head Neck Surg.* 2017;143(10):1032–1039

Vitamin D, Iron, and Zinc Supplementation

1. Baker RD, Greer FR; American Academy of Pediatrics Committee on Nutrition. Diagnosis and prevention of iron deficiency and iron-deficiency anemia in infants and young children (0–3 years of age). *Pediatrics.* 2010;126(5):1040–1050
2. Heinig MJ. Vitamin D and the breastfed infant: controversies and concerns. *J Hum Lact.* 2003;19(3):247–249
3. Heinig MJ, Brown KH, Lönnerdal B, Dewey KG. Zinc supplementation does not affect growth, morbidity, or motor development of US term breastfed infants at 4-10 mo of age. *Am J Clin Nutr.* 2006;84(3):594–601
4. Hollis BW, Wagner CL, Howard CR, et al. Maternal versus infant vitamin D supplementation during lactation: a randomized controlled trial. *Pediatrics.* 2015;136(4):625–634
5. Lawrence RA, Lawrence RM. *Breastfeeding: A Guide for the Medical Profession.* 8th ed. Philadelphia, PA: Elsevier; 2016
6. Perrine CG, Sharma AJ, Jefferds ME, Serdula MK, Scanlon KS. Adherence to vitamin D recommendations among US infants. *Pediatrics.* 2010;125(4):627–632
7. Wagner CL, Greer FR; American Academy of Pediatrics Section on Breastfeeding, Committee on Nutrition. Prevention of rickets and vitamin D deficiency in infants, children, and adolescents. *Pediatrics.* 2008;122(5):1142–1152
8. Ziegler EE, Nelson SE, Jeter JM. Vitamin D supplementation of breastfed infants: a randomized dose-response trial. *Pediatr Res.* 2014;76(2):177–183

Weaning

1. American Academy of Pediatrics. *New Mother's Guide to Breastfeeding.* Meek JY, ed. 3rd ed. New York, NY: Bantam Books; 2017
2. Huggins K, Ziedrich L. *The Nursing Mother's Guide to Weaning: How to Bring Breastfeeding to a Gentle Close, and How to Decide When the Time Is Right.* Rev ed. Boston, MA: Harvard Common Press; 2007
3. Lawrence RA, Lawrence RM. *Breastfeeding: A Guide for the Medical Profession.* 8th ed. Philadelphia, PA: Elsevier; 2016
4. Neifert M. *Great Expectations: The Essential Guide to Breastfeeding.*

Index

Page numbers in *italic* denote a photo (all photos are in color).